BEYOND ADVICE:

2. DEVELOPING MOTIVATIONAL SKILLS

Richard J. Botelho, BMedSci., B.M., B.S., MRCGP (UK)
Professor of Family Medicine and Nursing
Family Medicine Center, 885 South Avenue
Rochester, NY 14620, USA
Phone: (585) 442-7470, Ext. 508

Send suggestions for improving the next edition by going to:
www.MotivateHealthyHabits.com

Contents

To Eve, Anna, and Sara with love

Acknowledgments

I would like to thank Marlene Mussell and Ceil Goldman for their editorial support, Steve Marcus for his secretarial support, Hill Jason and Jane Westberg for their educational expertise, and my patients, students and professional colleagues, who contributed in countless different ways over many years.

Permission to Reproduce

Table 5a.10: Fagerstrom Test

Carfax Publishing Co. has given permission to adapt the Fagerstrom Test from Heatherton TF, Kozlowski LT, Frecker RC, et al. The Fagerstrom Test for Nicotine Dependence: A revision of the Fagerstrom Tolerance Questionnaire. British Journal of Addiction (1991); 86(9): 1119-1127.

PERSONAL INTRODUCTION

I am a British-trained general practitioner who has been teaching academic family medicine in the United States for 20 years. Over the past 8 years, I have done research and development in process improvement work on health behavior change. This work has focused on creating, testing and enhancing motivational innovations for educational and clinical purposes: changing practitioner and patient behavior to promote healthy habits and self-care of chronic diseases. This two-part book series, *Beyond Advice: 1. Becoming a Motivational Practitioner and 2. Developing Motivational Skills,* helps students and practitioners learn how to change their professional roles, assumptions and mental maps (Book 1) before developing the skills to help others (Book 2).This work is part of my never-ending journey of learning how to motivate healthy behaviors. I hope you may also consider embarking on a similar journey of lifelong learning, and contribute toward the advancement of this field.

In writing these books, I sought to compile and synthesize wisdom from multiple sources: patients, students, colleagues, health care practitioners, and expert educators, as well as from pragmatic approaches from different disciplines, selected theories and models, and a broad range of research evidence. This interdisciplinary approach to motivating behavior change goes beyond the current research evidence of randomized control trials to incorporate state-of-the-art practices. The major influences that have shaped the development of this approach are the Transtheoretical Model of Change (Jim Prochaska and Carlos DiClemente), Motivational Interviewing (William Miller and Steve Rollnick), Self-determination Theory (Ed Deci and Rich Ryan), Self-efficacy Theory (Albert Bandura), Relapse Prevention (Gordon Marlatt), and Solution-based Therapy (Steve De Shazer). My books build on the shoulders of these trail-blazers.

The magnitude of unhealthy behaviors in the general population is far too big for the health care system alone to treat everyone. Mutual Aid and Self-Help (MASH) approaches also are needed. Based on the above-mentioned books, I have written a MASH guidebook, *Motivate Healthy Habits: Change Yourself Before Helping Others,* to assist both you and your patients on an inner journey of self-directed change. This book taps into the most important yet underutilized resources: you, your family, and your friends all mobilizing to work on unhealthy behaviors.

These practitioner and lay books describe an integrated approach to helping professionals and the general public learn about motivating healthy habits. The Web site, www.MotivateHealthyHabits.com (under continual development), will also provide a place where you and your patients can share and learn from one another about motivating healthy habits. Visit this Web site to share stories, learn, get support, buy books for friends and family members, listen to audio, watch videos, or read book outlines for health care professionals. For wholesale prices for health and training organizations and bookstores, please send an e-mail to the address on the Web site.

INTRODUCTION TO THIS BOOK SERIES

Behavior change skills are fundamental core competencies for all health care practitioners. Yet, this topic is inadequately or poorly addressed in health care education. To promote health and prevent diseases due to unhealthy behaviors, we need to develop our motivational skills. However, the current challenge of helping patients to change their behaviors over time is even more difficult because health care training and delivery have become increasingly more complex and time-pressured. This raises a crucial question about how educational and health care organizations can help us enhance our motivational skills throughout our careers to improve the health of our patients. We need to address the discrepancies between the ideal behavior change and disease management programs and the realities of clinical practice. To work on this complex task, practitioners can use the following five-point strategy to achieve a long-range vision:

1. Enhance the quality of practitioner-patient interactions
   - Help practitioners recognize when behavioral interventions are ineffective and provide them with alternative ways of working with patients, so that clinical encounters are more productive.
   - Educate practitioners to use their limited time during patient encounters to deliver more potent, efficient and individualized interventions, so that their patients are more motivated to use their time effectively to work on behavior change between encounters.

2. Support ongoing professional and organizational development
   - Develop continuing professional development (CPD) approaches that help practitioners learn how to:
     o Change from the "fix-it," advice-giving role to the motivational role
     o Enhance their motivational skills over time
   - Develop comprehensive behavior change and disease management programs

3. Monitor organizational and practitioner performance
   - Develop the information technology support to gather data and analyze how the process of care improves patient outcomes at a population-based level, and provide ongoing feedback to practitioners and organizations.

4. Foster community mobilization
   - Encourage the general public to systematically use Mutual Aid and Self-Help (MASH) approaches to behavior change, with or without professional support

5. Advocate for changes in public policies
   - Encourage greater resource reallocation toward prevention, health promotion and disease management

This five-point strategy calls for public policy, community, organizational, practitioner and patient changes. Even with ideal public policies supporting this strategy, the patient is the ultimate determinant of the overall impact of any systematic approach. The quality of patient interactions and the effectiveness of individualized interventions will determine the ultimate success of any behavior change and disease management program. We cannot wait until such ideal public policies exist before we start to learn how to help patients change their unhealthy behaviors over time. To do more in less time in patient encounters (work smarter, not harder), we can begin by taking some time out from our already busy days to invest in learning new skills. This two-part practitioner book series, *Beyond Advice: 1. Becoming a Motivational Practitioner* and *Beyond Advice: 2. Developing Motivational Skills,* can help you with this long-term goal.

This book series goes beyond the current limits of traditional, evidence-based practice to incorporate:

- Experience-based approaches (narrative-based and qualitative methods)
- Motivational principles for overcoming the knowledge-behavior gap (e.g., I know what to do but don't do it) and for changing practitioner and patient behavior
- Nonlinear thinking (derived from systems, chaos and behavioral theories) to address cognitive-emotional dissonance (e.g., I think that I should change but don't feel like it) and the unpredictable, nonrational processes of change
- Continuous innovation, improvement and evaluation of developing and applying individualized interventions
- Continuing professional development precepts, involving practitioners creating and developing learning portfolios

All of these elements are applied to the challenge of motivating patients to change their unhealthy behaviors, with an emphasis on improving practitioner capabilities, skills and performance over time, not just competence. The underlying philosophy shaping this developmental process is influenced by the idea of building bridges between differing worldviews, rather than building from one particular professional worldview. To protect patients from the trappings of professional hegemony, this postmodern approach places a higher value on a bottom-up than a top-down practice, but without devaluing the contributions from theory-centric modernism and the research evidence generated from randomized controlled trials. This bottom-up perspective challenges the underlying assumptions of the modern but now traditional scientific approach. Proponents of this modernist approach might prematurely reject postmodernism, without appreciating the power of how these contrasting paradigms can complement one another.

Instead of imposing a theory-driven worldview on patients in research studies, we can begin to work from the patients' worldview and invite them to become the researchers of their own health, with us acting as co-investigators and researchers as our consultants. We use theories and models to fit into the patients' worlds rather than the other way around—making patients fit our theories. This postmodern approach places a higher emphasis on producing hard results in the complex, real world of practice, rather than on generating hard evidence that can be discovered in the controlled, decontextualized world of research. In contrast, the traditional scientific approach places a higher emphasis on generating hard evidence at the expense of producing hard results— creating a chasm between research and practice. This gap has led to the development of the term "translational research": a term that is fundamentally flawed because it refers to a predominantly one-way process from research to practice, as opposed to a two-way, collaborative process. It is like building a bridge from only the research side of the river. This book series begins a process of building a bridge from both the research and practice sides, and invites the reader to improve the ongoing process of advancing the field of behavior change. These books will be episodically updated and improved by incorporating ongoing input from multiple perspectives (patients, family members, students, practitioners, and researchers), based on the experiences of working in different contexts and cultures. Any comments you have to improve the books and their use with patients will be appreciatively received.

Consider using this book series as part of your own continuing professional development process, whether or not you are using it in conjunction with a formal course or curriculum. These two books give equal importance to learning about:

- Improving your own health behaviors
- Exploring your professional role and assumptions
- Developing your motivational skills

Learning how to change yourself (personally and professionally) as you learn how to develop motivational skills will help you become a more effective and efficient motivational practitioner. Discover the extent to which this premise, changing yourself facilitates motivating change in others, holds true for you.

Book 1 outlines a six-step approach for motivating health behavior change, so that you can learn more about developing individualized interventions to meet patients' changing needs over time. You can apply this approach to all unhealthy behaviors. If you learn how to counsel patients with one unhealthy behavior (e.g., tobacco use), you will learn more quickly how to counsel patients with any other unhealthy behaviors. **Book 2** will help you learn how to initiate "change" dialogues with patients, so that you can develop the art of engaging patients in such dialogues over time. To work on this lifelong learning goal, you can develop a learning plan to enhance your motivational skills throughout your career, whatever your level of experience and competence. In addition, you can gather evidence about how your plan contributed to your continuing professional development and improved patient outcomes.

In spite of the high prevalence of unhealthy behaviors, most educational programs do not adequately prepare us for working with patients on these issues over time; we are left to learn on the job. Throughout our training and careers, we can use a variety of on-going learning opportunities, educational methods and developmentally appropriate activities to enhance our motivational skills: self-directed learning (as described in *Beyond Advice: Developing Motivational Skills*); Web-based instruction (www.MotivateHealthyHabits.com); longitudinal skills-based training opportunities in small groups led by supervisors or facilitators; direct observation with simulated and actual patients with feedback and evaluation; and, in-depth learning experiences working with a small number of patients on behavior change over 1-2 years. A cascade of positive benefits can accrue from using such continuing professional development methods:

- Reduce your frustration in working with so-called "resistant" patients
- Enjoy engaging patients in dialogues about change over time
- Develop individualized approaches to meet patients' changing needs over time
- Enhance patients' readiness to change
- Improve patient outcomes

This book series describes several models to enhance your ability to work with patients. Once you have learned about these different models, you can shift from being focused on learning models to enhancing your ability to work in patient-centered ways.

Do not quench your inspiration and your imagination;
do not become the slave of your model.
Vincent Van Gogh (1853-1890)

May this precept sustain your enthusiasm and inspire your creativity to work on the challenges of helping patients change over time.

GUIDE TO THIS BOOK

To develop an effective lifelong learning plan, it is worthwhile reflecting about this question:

> *To what extent did your training and education prepare you*
> *for lifelong learning in how to motivate patients to change?*

Your training and educational programs (current or past) can disable or enable your continuing professional development at motivating patients to change. Brief descriptions of such programs are provided next to help you reflect further about this question.

A. Training Program

Trainers focus on acculturating trainees to a particular set of beliefs, values, and attitudes: "This is the way things are done." Such professional socialization or indoctrination indicates an inward focus: a preoccupation with, and a group loyalty toward, the building of a particular worldview. Such group behavior is motivated by positive and negative reasons. Positive reasons include: passionate investment in a particular worldview, theory, or model; excitement about doing pioneer work at the cutting edge of medical science; and the quest for new behavioral or psychological interventions within a particular model or school of thought.

Negative reasons include: the imposition of a worldview, theory, or model to the exclusion of others; individual insecurities that coalesce to form insular groups; and dysfunctional leadership arising from unrecognized needs for dominance and control. Professional groups with a predominance of negative reasons are intolerant of deviations from their norm. They foster a loyalty toward the ascendancy of their work rather than toward the best interests of patients or the health of a population. They are well defended against challenges to their professional mores and practices. Furthermore, trainees who challenge group norms risk marginalization, exclusion, and even rejection.

B. Educational Program

When educators encourage learners to challenge the status quo of group norms and their implicit assumptions, they promote an openness in exploring new, contrasting, or even contradictory perspectives. They also provide flexible training and educational methods to promote professional development, differentiation, and diversity. This process can help practitioners learn more about other worldviews as well as better understand how their own worldview affects their work with others. A value is given both to building bridges between practitioners' and patients' worldviews, and to uncovering what is behind patients' stories about their risk behaviors. Effective education prepares practitioners to work with patients to discuss their differences in perceptions and values about risk behaviors. To work in a population-based manner, practitioners are trained to work in interdisciplinary teams.

Such an educational process encourages you to reflect critically about your learning experiences so that you can work more effectively with patients over time. You devote more effort and loyalty toward enhancing patient care outcomes than toward a particular school of thought, theory, training method, or the self-interest of your professional group.

C. Comparing Programs

A crucial distinction between these two approaches needs highlighting because it can make an enormous difference in your ability to develop as a lifelong learner. Training programs are theory-centered or centered on a particular model. An exclusive reliance on a particular theory or training model can foster a rigid "method-centeredness" that can block practitioners from learning how to develop as a lifelong learner. In contrast, educational programs emphasize what works for an individual patient using whatever method, theory, or model seems appropriate: in other words, it aspires to be patient-centered.

CONTINUING PROFESSIONAL DEVELOPMENT

A continuing professional development (CPD) curriculum on motivating health behavior change must revisit topics at increasing levels of complexity to foster lifelong learning, enrich professional development, and improve clinical performance. Such a curriculum helps practitioners develop their skills at self-directed learning as well as provide opportunities for small group learning, individual supervision, Web-based training, and/or mentorship throughout their formal education and their careers. Given that such ideal curricula are rare, it becomes even more important to create your own lifelong learning plan for developing motivational skills. A CPD model has been developed to assist you with this learning process. This model consist of four phases:

- Self-focused—analyze your health behaviors and professional role
- Method-focused—learn about the six-step approach
- Learner-centered—identify your strengths and weaknesses
- Patient-centered—learn about developing individualized interventions

Using this model as a guide, you first begin with a self-analysis about professional roles and personal behaviors before using a method-focused approach to select the skills that you want to practice and develop. Once you have learned one set of skills, then you can learn another.

As you begin to identify your strengths and weaknesses, you can enhance your strengths and rectify your weaknesses to enhance your range and depth of skills. This is being learner-centered. After mastering a range of skills, you can select and test options that you think would be most helpful for an individual patient. This is being patient-centered. Learning how to motivate behavior change is a lifelong process; your learning needs will change throughout your career. Even if you are an experienced and seasoned practitioner, you will be new at developing some interpersonal skills, but your past experience may enable you to acquire new skills more quickly than when you were a trainee. On the other hand, some experienced practitioners are slower than trainees in developing new skills because of training-of-origin issues; they have developed habits that run counter to the new approach. In effect, their old mental map creates roadblocks in learning how to use a new mental map; they have to unlearn old habits before developing new ones.

Both experienced practitioners and trainees face similar issues when they develop new skills: vulnerability, awkwardness and/or fear of risk-taking. An element of emotional reactivity (excitement, anxiety, humor, tension, or fun) is needed to create vivid, emotionally charged events that will imprint your learning experiences, so that they can have lasting positive effects on your professional behavior.

HOW TO USE THIS BOOK

Whatever your level of clinical experience, you can use this book to create your own learning plan and portfolio in how to become a more effective and efficient motivational practitioner. This process involves learning how to initiate and engage patients in "change" dialogues over time. Dialogues about health behavior change go beyond the traditional, one-way question and answer clinical interviews toward a more flexible practitioner-patient partnership.

This book uses a learner-centered approach to help you clarify your educational needs. The worksheets in Chapter 1 can help you to self-assess your educational needs and to develop your learning plan: set specific goals and select methods to meet those goals. As you progress, you can create a learning portfolio to provide ongoing evidence about how your educational and clinical experiences contribute toward improving your competence and performance. (In addition, examples of such plans and portfolios will be downloadable from the Web site www.MotivateHealthyHabits.com.). Ideally, your learning plan should fit in with your organizational plan for developing behavior change and disease management programs in your practice setting.

You can use the improvement cycle over and over again as part of the process of applying the continuing professional development (CPD) model. The outcomes in applying this CPD model are as follows:

- Self-focused—change your own health behaviors and professional role
- Method-focused—use the micro skills in the six-step model
- Learner-centered—enhance your range and depth of skills
- Patient-centered—help patients become more ready to change

To prepare yourself for becoming a motivational practitioner, you can use this book to develop self-focused and method-focused learning goals. To enhance your range and depth of motivational skills, you can use the companion book to develop method-focused, learner-centered and patient-centered learning goals. Chapter 1 in *Beyond Advice: 1. Developing Motivational Skills* provides guidance on how you can conduct self-assessments on the four phases of this CPD model. You can assess the impact of reading these books on your level of understanding about—and your competence in applying—key concepts and models, motivational principles and a wide range of micro skills. This process can help you refine your learning goals over time.

Each person is unique in what helps him or her change. This book offers a wide range of options for helping you initiate constructive dialogues with your patients. The K.I.S.S. precept (keep it simple and sophisticated) can help you learn how to individualize your approach with patients in order to meet their changing needs over time. The motivational principles (described in Chapter 1 of Book 1) can help guide you in how to engage patients effectively in ongoing dialogues about change. Your learning plan can help you refine the art of dialogue with patients about behavior change throughout your career. When you get stuck in working with patients, you can review sections of this book to give you some ideas about how to overcome these impasses. With time and practice, you will expand your repertoire of motivational skills.

An Overview of What You Could Learn
    Section I describes how you can design a learning plan: set your learning goals (Chapter 1), select educational methods (Chapter 2), and create a learning portfolio to document your progress toward your goals (Chapter 3).

    Section II addresses three health behaviors. Chapters 4a, 5a and 6a describe key findings and specific issues about excessive alcohol use, tobacco use, and self-care of diabetes respectively, because these behaviors raise different issues even though you can use a similar process for motivating health behavior change. For example, nicotine addiction prevents many smokers from quitting. A key issue is to assess the severity of patients' addiction and their need for nicotine replacement therapy, in addition to motivating patients to set a quit date. In contrast, alcohol presents different issues. Most patients who drink above low-risk limits do not have evidence of alcohol abuse and dependency, which can create diagnostic uncertainty when addressing this topic. Diabetic self-care raises the issue of patients dealing with multiple tasks due to multiple-risk behaviors, so you need to negotiate an agenda with them and let them set priorities and select the goals for change.

Chapters 4b, 5b, and 6b discuss how you can initiate constructive dialogues about these three health behaviors in busy, time-pressured work environments, such as primary care and hospital settings. Chapter 4b (Reducing Alcohol Risk and Harm) provides greater detail than Chapters 5b (Helping Resistant Smokers to Quit) and 6b (Facilitating Self-care of Diabetes) because the alcohol and drug field has produced the most motivational approaches to behavior change.

In the spirit of this book, adapt your educational methods to suit your changing educational needs over time so that you can enhance your range and depth of motivational skills and individualize your learning plan for continuing professional development. Select options and discover what works for both you and your patients. This book may help stimulate your curiosity about working with patients and enhance your professional commitment to promoting healthy behaviors. Such commitment will not only enhance your professional satisfaction but also improve your effectiveness in helping patients change.

An Interdisciplinary Note

The term "practitioner" is used to describe all professionals who help patients to change: physicians, physician assistants, nurse practitioners, nurses, psychologists, therapists, community and public health workers, social workers, and allied health professionals. All members of your health care team can benefit from learning about how to become motivational practitioners and can adopt a variety of roles when working with patients. Practitioners adopting either a fix-it, preventive, or motivational role are given the following abbreviations: FP, PP, or MP, while physicians are more specifically identified as Dr. F., Dr. P., or Dr. M. The text is written in the first person (we) and third person (you) to describe the fix-it and motivational role respectively. I hope that this will create a tone that engages you in a process of professional change in ways that you may replicate with your patients in motivating positive behavior change.

SECTION I

DESIGN YOUR LEARNING PLAN

To design your learning plan, you can use a continuing professional development model (CPD) and the worksheets provided in Chapter 1 to assess your level of competence and clarify your educational needs. This process can help you set your learning goals. You can then select appropriate educational methods (Chapter 2) to work on your goals and create a portfolio (Chapter 3) to reinforce your learning and to monitor your progress over time.

CHAPTER 1

SET YOUR LEARNING GOALS

FOR REFLECTION

*How can you set your learning goals to foster
your continuing professional development?*

OVERVIEW

A continuing professional development (CPD) model can help you design a learning plan for enhancing your motivational skills over time. This model consists of four phases:

- **Self-focused**—analyze your health behaviors, professional roles and assumptions
- **Method-focused**—learn the micro skills in the six-step approach
- **Learner-centered**—identify your strengths and weaknesses to improve your skills
- **Patient-centered**—develop individualized interventions for your patients

Self-assessment worksheets are provided to help you clarify your educational needs and set goals (small or large, short-term or long-term) for each phase of the CPD model. You can use the PARE improvement cycle to work on achieving your goals.

To foster lifelong learning in helping patients change over time, you can move back and forth between these phases throughout your career, depending on your evolving educational needs and learning goals.

SET YOUR LEARNING GOALS

A framework for understanding the incompetence-competence continuum can help to clarify your educational needs and the need to set learning goals.

- Unconsciously incompetent—You are unaware of what you need to know in terms of developing new skills.
- Consciously incompetent—You are aware of what you do not know and what micro skills you need to develop. This process can help you clarify your educational needs and set priorities about your learning goals.
- Consciously competent—You consciously use your skills and are aware of your profile in terms of professional competence. You can develop an individualized learning plan of goals to enhance your overall profile of skills, improving your strengths and addressing your weaknesses.
- Unconsciously competent—You unconsciously use your skills automatically without full awareness of how effective you are.

This chapter provides worksheets for helping you become more aware of your level of professional competence and your educational needs. The worksheets provide a comprehensive list of skills, and you may be at different places for different categories of skills. For example, one student was not fully aware of her natural ability to establish empathic relationships with patients (unconsciously competent), but was consciously aware of her difficulties in implementing a plan with her patients (consciously incompetent). Another student had a natural ability to implement plans with his patients, but he was not aware of his limitations in developing empathic relationships with his patients.

Worksheets 1.1-1.9 can help you become aware of the micro skills that you need to learn about, so you can begin to set learning goals, as well as become aware of how unconsciously competent you are in using specific skills. Even then, you can assess your level of your competence and set even higher goals for improvement. You can use as little or as much of the worksheets as you like at any one time, and revisit them in ways that best suit your changing needs and preferences over time.

Because you can use these worksheets to self-assess your level of competence in using a wide range of micro skills, they can help you become more aware of your profile of professional competence and educational needs. This process can help you begin to work on the first part of designing your individualized learning plan: set your learning goals (short term and long term). As you improve, you will refine your goals over time, depending on your changing needs. You select appropriate educational methods (described in Chapter 2 of this book) to achieve your goals. Such a learning plan can help you enhance your ability to act as a catalytic agent for change. This plan can have a cascade of positive short-term and long-term effects on you and your patients by:

- Reducing your frustration in dealing with resistant, indifferent, and ambivalent patients
- Enhancing your competence and professional satisfaction in working with these patients
- Enhancing the quality of dialogue and partnerships with your patients
- Helping patients become more ready for change
- Improving your clinical performance in terms of patient outcomes

Only you, however, can decide whether these promises hold true for you. To assess the impact of your learning plan on you and your patients, it is vitally important to gather ongoing evidence for your learning portfolio, because otherwise it can be very difficult to assess what improvements you are making over time.[1-5] This critical issue will be revisited in Chapter 3, but the first task is to learn how to set learning goals for developing and enhancing your skills, using a continuing professional development model.

USING PARE IMPROVEMENT CYCLES IN A CPD MODEL

Kolb's learning cycle and the PDSA (Prepare, Do, Study, Act) improvement cycle have influenced the development of the PARE improvement cycle: Prepare, Act, Reflect, and Enhance.[6;7]

- **Prepare**—Clarify your educational needs and set goals. Prepare to achieve your goals: for example, select appropriate educational methods and resources.
- **Act**—Use educational methods to achieve your goals. Increase your knowledge and/or put new understanding into action.
- **Reflect**—Assess whether these educational methods helped you achieve your goals.[8;9] Ask others to assess the extent to which you achieve your goals.[10]
- **Enhance**—Generate ideas about how to improve what you did. Ask others for new ideas, and use these new ideas in your next improvement cycle.

To work toward your goals, you can use the PARE cycle over and over again within each phase of the CPD model. A model of this interaction is shown in Figure 1.1 on the next page.

Figure 1.1:—A Model for Continuing Professional Development Using PARE Improvement Cycles

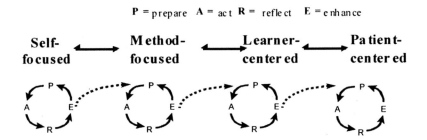

P = prepare **A** = act **R** = reflect **E** = enhance

CLARIFYING YOUR EDUCATIONAL NEEDS

The CPD model provides a framework for lifelong learning that can help you decide where to focus your time and energy. You can use Worksheets 1.1-1.9 to conduct a self-assessment for the first three phases of the CPD model; analyze your health behaviors, your professional role, your level of understanding about motivational principles, your ability to address different health behaviors, and your range and depth of motivational skills. This process can help you clarify your educational needs and set learning goals. During your career, you can move back and forth between these phases and use the PARE improvement cycles repeatedly, depending on your evolving learning goals. These worksheets can help you to set small or large, short-term or long-term goals for each phase.

After working on your goals, you can score the items on the worksheets again and make notes for your learning portfolio on the reasons for changing your scores. Self-assessment, however, is subject to many potential biases. For example, if you tend to rate yourself as having high self-efficacy, you are more likely to give yourself higher scores than someone who has a low self-efficacy. While it is important to reflect and even make notes about these potential biases, the process of scoring yourself again at a later date can help to decide whether and how you are making any progress in your professional development. The process of writing down your reasons for the changes in your scores provides qualitative data about how you are making progress in your professional development. To validate your self-assessment, you can ask for opinions from third party (patient, peer or expert consultant) about how you perceive yourself in comparison to how others perceive you.

A. Self-focused Goals

The internal process of learning how to change your own health behaviors and how to become a motivational practitioner can accelerate the external process of expanding your depth and range of motivational skills to help others change. This option, however, can be threatening for some people, seem irrelevant or unnecessary to others, or even evoke resistance in still others to facing their own health behaviors or exploring the kind of professional role that they adopt with patients. Thus, even if this option makes perfect rational sense to you, you may have a mixture of positive and negative responses and feelings about this idea. Whatever your internal reaction, it is worth reflecting about what makes you approach or avoid the options of exploring personal and professional issues about self-change.

You can use Worksheet 1.1a to analyze your health behaviors and your readiness to change them. This process can help you set some goals for changing one of your own health behaviors. You can use Worksheet 1.1b to rate your level of understanding about the differences in professional roles and your competence to act as a motivational practitioner. This process can help you set some learning goals about professional change.

WORKSHEET 1.1a: SELF-FOCUSED GOALS (health behaviors)

Develop a learning plan about changing your health behaviors.

Assess some issues about your health behaviors using the checklist below. Circle a response to each health decision using the letter code N or Y.

N = not applicable to me.
Y = yes. For each yes response, circle the "readiness-to-change" scale:

1 = not thinking about change, 2 = thinking about change, 3 = preparing to change

Self-assessment of your health behaviors	Response		Readiness to change		
1. I do not exercise enough	N	Y	1	2	3
2. I have unhealthy eating habits	N	Y	1	2	3
3. I am overweight	N	Y	1	2	3
4. I do not put on my seat belt in my car every time	N	Y	1	2	3
5. I sometimes forget to take prescription drugs	N	Y	1	2	3
6. I do not practice safe sex every time	N	Y	1	2	3
7. I sometimes forget to use contraception	N	Y	1	2	3
8. I use tobacco products	N	Y	1	2	3
9. I drink alcohol more than					
For men: 14 drinks per week	N	Y	1	2	3
For women: 7 drinks per week	N	Y	1	2	3
10. I use illegal drugs	N	Y	1	2	3

Make some note about your readiness to change.

_____

_____

_____

_____

Based on your self-assessment, write down some learning goals.

_____

_____

_____

_____

WORKSHEET 1.1b: SELF-FOCUSED GOALS (roles)

Develop a learning plan for understanding professional roles.

Assess your understanding about professional roles before and after reading Chapters 2 and 3 in Book 1, *Beyond Advice: Becoming a Motivational Practitioner.*

Rate your level of understanding (u-score) about professional roles, using this 0-10 scale:

0	1	2	3	4	5	6	7	8	9	10
None					*Moderate*					*Very High*

Assess your understanding about the differences between the fix-it and motivational roles in terms of: *fill in date*	*U-score*	*U-score*
Overall role characteristics		
Role functions		
Role boundaries		
Role outcomes		
Assess your level of competence (C-score) in: *fill in date*	*C-score*	*C-score*
Adopting a motivational role		

Write down your reasons for your scores before reading Chapters 2 and 3 in Book 1. After reading the chapters, write down your reasons for changes in your scores.

_____

_____

_____

_____

_____

Based on what you have written, consider writing down some learning goals.

_____

_____

_____

B. Method-focused Issues

An understanding of motivational principles and the six-step micro skills approach may help you learn how to become a motivational practitioner. These steps are:

Six-step Approach
1. Building Partnerships
2. Negotiating an Agenda
3. Assessing Resistance and Motivation
4. Enhancing Mutual Understanding
5. Implementing a Plan for Change
6. Following Through

You can use Worksheets 1.2a and 1.2b to rate your level of understanding about motivational principles and the six-step approach before and after reading Chapters 1 and 8 in Book 1, and later, after you have begun to use these principles and this approach with patients. The learning process may help you address:

- Self-focused issues in terms of helping you internalize motivational principles and the six-step approach.
- Learner-centered issues in terms of overcoming the particular challenges that you encounter in applying motivational principles and the six-step approach in practice, and in using specific micro skills with patients.

To become more familiar with some of the micro skills used in the six-step approach, you can watch a demonstration of the three sequential goals listed below on a CD-ROM or videotape and at the Web site www.MotivateHealthyhabits.com/intro. This observational process can help you better understand how to use a limited range of micro skills:

- Clarify a patient's issues about change
- Lower patient resistance
- Enhance patient motivation

Appendix A describes how to complete these three tasks, using the micro skills to address tobacco cessation. You can use the checklists to assess your level of understanding in employing these micro skills before and watching these demonstrations.

WORKSHEET 1.2a: METHOD-FOCUSED GOALS

Develop a learning plan to better understand motivational principles.
Assess your understanding of these principles before and after reading Book 1.

Use this scale to rate your understanding of motivational principles:

0	1	2	3	4	5	6	7	8	9	10
None					*Moderate*					*Very High*

How would you rate your understanding of these principles? Fill in dates	*U-score*	*U-score*
Develop empathic relationships		
Clarify roles and responsibilities for behavior change		
Respect patients' autonomy: use influence, not control		
Gain consent from patients to address behavior change		
Work at a pace sensitive to patients' needs and their readiness to change		
Help patients explore and understand their values and perceptions		
Help patients decide whether to change their values and perceptions		
Focus on strengths and health, rather than on weaknesses and pathology		
Focus on solutions rather than on problems		
Enhance patients' confidence and ability to change		
Negotiate reasonable goals for change		
Help patients believe healthy outcomes are possible		
Help patients increase their supports and reduce their barriers to change		
Help patients develop plans to prevent relapse		

Write down your reasons for your scores before reading Book 1. After reading this book, write down your reasons for any change in your scores.

_____

_____

_____

_____

Based on what you have written, consider writing down some learning goals.

_____

_____

WORKSHEET 1.2b: METHOD-FOCUSED GOALS

Develop a learning plan to better understand the six-step approach.
Assess your understanding before and after reading Chapter 8 in Book 1.

How would you rate your understanding of the six-step approach, using the 0-10 scale? *fill in dates*	*U-score*	*U-score*
1. Building partnerships		
2. Negotiating an agenda		
3. Assessing resistance and motivation		
4. Enhancing mutual understanding		
5. Implementing a plan		
6. Following through		

Write down your reasons for your scores before reading Chapter 8 in Book 1. After reading this chapter, write down your reasons for any change in your scores.

_____

_____

_____

_____

_____

_____

Based on what you have written, consider writing down some learning goals.

_____

_____

_____

_____

C. Learner-centered Issues

Your level of experience may or may not relate to your level of competence. Experienced but poorly trained practitioners may still feel incompetent in addressing behavior change; conversely, some well-trained yet inexperienced practitioners may yet feel competent in this area. Whatever your experience level, a structured approach to learning a new method can help you systematically develop these skills more efficiently than learning from "trial-and-error" clinical experience. To consider learner-centered issues, you can begin by assessing your level of experience and competence in addressing different health behaviors and using specific micro skills.

1. Analyze your ability to address different health behaviors.

Worksheet 1.3 can help you rate your initial level of competence (C-score) in addressing different health behaviors. You can reassess yourself later to monitor your progress. As you learn more, you may realize that you know less (or more) about motivating a certain behavior change than you thought, and you may even rate your competence score lower (or higher) than you did the first time you filled in the checklist. Your changes in scores is much less important than what you discover in thinking about *why* you changed your score. Document and discuss these changes with others.

WORKSHEET 1.3: LEARNER-CENTERED GOALS

Develop some learning goals to enhance your ability for addressing different behaviors.

Assess your level of competence (C-score), using the 0-10 scale to fill in the table below.

0	1	2	3	4	5	6	7	8	9	10
None					*Moderate*					*Very High*

Assess Your Level of Competence

How would you rate C-score in helping patients to: *fill in dates*	*C-score before reading Book 1*	*C-score after reading Book 1*	*C-score after practice sessions*
Quit smoking			
Quit alcohol or reduce intake			
Improve self-care of diabetes			
Lose weight			
Increase exercise level			
Practice safe sex			
Stop using illegal drugs			
Prevent unplanned pregnancies			
Take medications as recommended			
Motivate health behaviors overall			

Look over your notes you made while reading Book 1. Write down your reasons for your initial scores.

_____

_____

Based on your self-assessment, write down some learning goals.

_____

_____

At a later date, make notes for the reasons about the changes in your scores

_____

2. Develop learning goals to enhance your skills.

Chapters 9-14 in *Beyond Advice: Becoming a Motivational Practitioner* describe each step of the six-step approach in detail. Or, you can read Chapters 4b, 5b or 6b in this book to familiarize yourself with the labels that describe the different micro skills. Such preparatory reading can help you fill in Worksheets 1.4-1.9 (covering each of the six steps) to rate your overall level of skills. This process can also help you develop your learning goals. Start with a limited number of goals focusing on specific micro skills. You can use the worksheets again to assess the impact of your practice sessions on improving your competence in this area. Think of each worksheet as a collection of building blocks to construct a foundation for lifelong learning.

Over time, you can learn the micro skills used in the six-step approach and develop a profile of your strengths and weaknesses. You can then decide how to enhance your strengths and rectify your weaknesses. To expand your range and depth of skills, you will need to practice specific skills in role plays or in patient encounters. Ideally, this kind of learning is enhanced when you can debrief about these interactions (personal recall, tape recorded or videotaped role plays/patient encounters) with peers, colleagues, facilitators, supervisors, and/or expert coaches. The focus of these discussions is on how these activities can enhance your overall skills without focusing at this point on their clinical impact on patients.

For example, some practitioners are very effective at supporting patients to explore and better understand their values and perceptions about behavior change, without implying that they need to make a decision about change; in other words, they are good at being nondirect with patients. On the other hand, they have difficulties with being direct with them. Conversely, some practitioners are very effective at helping patients challenge themselves to address behavior change; in other words, they are good at being direct with patients and help patients decide whether to change their values and perceptions about behavior change. On the other hand, they have difficulties with being nondirect with patients. Both kinds of practitioners need to learn how to rectify their weaknesses and thereby expand their range of skills to learn how best to work with patients over time.

WORKSHEET 1.4
ENHANCE YOUR PARTNERSHIP-BUILDING SKILLS

After reading Chapters 9a, 9b and 9c in Book 1 or the relevant sections in Chapters 4b, 5b or 6b in this book, use the 0-10 scale to rate your level of competence (C-score).

0	1	2	3	4	5	6	7	8	9	10
None					*Moderate*					*Very High*

How would you rate your C-score?	After some reading preparation	After a practice session
Develop empathic skills *a. Use open-ended questions*		
b. Use reflective listening		
c. Paraphrase		
d. Validate feelings		
e. Normalize behaviors		
f. Affirm strengths		
g. Use probing questions		
Use relational skills *a. Put patient in the one-up position*		
b. Take the one-down position		
Clarify roles and responsibilities		

Look over your notes that you made while reading Chapters 9a, 9b and 9c. Write down your reasons for your initial scores.

_____

_____

Based on your self-assessment, write down some learning goals.

_____

_____

Make notes about whether your practice session helped you to improve your scores.

_____

_____

WORKSHEET 1.5
ENHANCE YOUR AGENDA-SETTING SKILLS

After reading Chapter 10 in Book 1 and the relevant sections in Chapters 4b, 5b or 6b in this book, use the 0-10 scale to rate your level of competence (C-score).

0	1	2	3	4	5	6	7	8	9	10
None					*Moderate*					*Very High*

How would you rate your C-score?	*After some reading preparation*	*After a practice session*
Prevention-focused approach *a. Consent-gaining, direct questions*		
b. Leading questions		
c. Prefacing statements		
Problem-focused approach *a. Prefacing statements*		
b. Exploratory questions		
c. Leading questions		

Look over your notes that you made while reading Chapter 10 in Book 1 and the relevant sections in Chapters 4b, 5b or 6b in this book. Write down your reasons for your initial scores.

_____

_____

_____

Based on your self-assessment, write down some learning goals.

_____

_____

_____

Make notes about whether your practice session helped you to improve your scores.

_____

_____

_____

WORKSHEET 1.6
ENHANCE YOUR SKILLS AT ASSESSING RESISTANCE AND MOTIVATION

After reading Chapter 11 in Book 1 and the relevant sections in Chapters 4b, 5b or 6b in this book, use the 0-10 scale to rate your level of competence (C-score).

0	1	2	3	4	5	6	7	8	9	10
None					*Moderate*					*Very High*

How would you rate your C-score?	*After some reading preparation*	*After a practice session*
Ask about readiness to change		
Provide a stage-specific rationale for using the decision balance		
Use a decision balance with a patient		
Explain "think" and "feeling" score for resistance and motivation		
Assess motives for change		
Assess competing priorities and energy		
Assess confidence and ability to change		
Assess supports and barriers		

Look over your notes that you made while reading Chapter 11 in Book 1. Write down your reasons for your initial scores.

_____

_____

_____

Based on your self-assessment, write down some learning goals.

_____

_____

Make notes about whether your practice session helped you to improve your scores.

_____

_____

WORKSHEET 1.7
ENHANCE YOUR SKILLS IN DEVELOPING MUTUAL UNDERSTANDING

After reading Chapter 12 in Book 1 and the relevant sections in Chapters 4b, 5b or 6b in this book, use the 0-10 scale to rate your level of competence (C-Score).

0	1	2	3	4	5	6	7	8	9	10
None					*Moderate*					*Very High*

How would you rate your C-score?	*After some reading preparation*	*After a practice session*
Educate about the need for behavior change in a patient-centered way		
Use nondirect interventions		
a. Probe priorities		
b. Use double-sided reflection		
c. Explore the future		
d. Acknowledge ambivalence		
e. Emphasize personal responsibility/choice		
f. Use simple reflection		
Use direct interventions		
a. Use back-to-the future questioning		
b. Use benefit substitution		
c. Clarify values		
d. Challenge rationalizations		
e. Use discrepancies		
f. Reframe items, issues or events		
g. Challenge claims or positions		
h. Use differences in motivational reasons		
Clarify differences in perceptions about confidence and ability to change		

Look over your notes that you made while reading Chapter 12 in Book 1. Write down your reasons for your initial scores.

_____

_____

Based on your self-assessment, write down some learning goals.

_____

_____

Make notes about whether your practice session helped you to improve your scores.

WORKSHEET 1.8
ENHANCE YOUR SKILLS AT IMPLEMENTING A PLAN

After reading Chapter 13 in Book 1 and/or the relevant sections in Chapters 4b, 5b or 6b in this book, use the 0-10 scale to rate your level of competence (C-score).

0	1	2	3	4	5	6	7	8	9	10
None					Moderate					Very High

How would you rate your C-score?	After some reading preparation	After a practice session
Evaluate patient commitment (competing priorities, energy and motives)		
Decide about goals a. Practitioner-selected goals		
b. Patient-selected goals		
c. Negotiated approach to goal setting		
Set a goal for change a. Think more about quitting		
b. Prepare for a change		
c. Set a quit date		
d. Additional options		
Clarify persistent differences in perceptions		
Use solution-based approaches		

Look over your notes that you made while reading Chapter 13 in Book 1. Write down your reasons for your initial scores.

_____

_____

Based on your self-assessment, write down some learning goals

_____

_____

Make notes about whether your practice session helped you to improve your scores.

_____

WORKSHEET 1.9
ENHANCE YOUR SKILLS AT FOLLOWING THROUGH

After reading Chapter 14 in Book 1 and the relevant sections in Chapters 4b, 5b or 6b in this book, use the 0-10 scale to rate your level of competence (C-score).

0	1	2	3	4	5	6	7	8	9	10
None					*Moderate*					*Very High*

How would you rate your C-score?	*After some reading preparation*	*After a practice session*
Provide rationale for follow-up		
Clarify patient's reason for follow-up		
Arrange follow-up		
Use methods to assure change		
a. A diary to track change		
b. Relapse prevention approach		
Management of risk situations		
Pharmacological management		
Emotional management		
Reevaluation of supports		
Reevaluation of barriers		
Use of positive reinforcement		
c. Motivational reevaluation		

Look over your notes that you made while reading Chapter 14 in Book 1 and the relevant sections in Chapters 4b, 5b or 6b in this book. Write down your reasons for your initial scores.

_____

_____

Based on your self-assessment, write down some learning goals.

_____

_____

_____

Make notes about whether your practice session helped you to improve your scores.

_____

Chapter 2 can help you select educational methods to work on achieving your learning goals. After practicing these skills, you can reflect about performance and score yourself again. As suggested in Chapter 3 in this book, you can make notes about why you changed your scores for your learning portfolio.

D. Patient-centered Issues

Once you have mastered a range of skills, you can use patient-centered approaches. You will practice how to work in a highly individualized manner with patients in order to have a positive impact in helping them work through the change process. You will encounter "stuck moments" with some patients and challenges in working with patients over time. (See Chapter 2, page 42, for a discussion of bail-out strategies to use in such moments.) These kinds of experiences can help you identify your particular difficulties in working effectively in a patient-centered way. You can take advantage of these learning opportunities if you can debrief soon after these interactions (using personal recall, audiotaped or videotaped encounters) with patients, peers, colleagues, facilitators, supervisors, and/or expert coaches. Such discussions can clarify whether, how and why you are being effective in working in patient-centered ways. For example, to what extent are you being effectively direct and nondirect during the course of your dialogue with a patient? This process can help you develop a patient-centered learning plan that identifies your particular goals for improvement.

Reflect and Enhance
In what ways have this chapter and Worksheets 1.1-1.9 helped you learn how to:
- *Assess your level of competence and clarify your educational needs*
- *Develop learning goals based on this self-assessment*

How will this new learning help you enhance the process of designing your learning plan?

MOVING ON

This chapter can help you design the initial part of your learning plan. Worksheets 1.1–1.9 can help you to conduct self-assessments and to develop your learning goals. To complete your learning plan, the next chapter will describe different educational methods for helping you work toward your goals.

Reference List
1. Challis M, Mathers NJ, Howe AC, et al. Portfolio-based learning: continuing medical education for general practitioners—a mid-point evaluation. Med Educ 1997;31: 22-26
2. Department of Health. A Review of Continuing Professional Development in General Practice. 1998
3. Snadden D, Thomas M. Portfolio learning in general practice vocational training—does it work? Medical Education 1998;32: 401-406

4. Challis MC. Portfolio based learning and assessment in medical education. (AMEE Medical Education Guide No. 11 (revised). Medical Teacher 1999;221: 370-386

5. Snadden D, Thomas M. AME Guide No. 11: The use of portfolio learning in medical education. Medical Teacher 1998;30: 192-199

6. Kolb DA. Experiential Learning. Chicago: Prentice Hall; 1984

7. Langley GJ, Nolan KM, Nolan TW, et al. The improvement guide: A practical approach to enhancing organizational performance. San Francisco, CA: Jossey-Bass; 1996

8. Boud D, Keogh R, Walker D. Reflection: Turning Experience Into Learning. London: Kogan Page; 1985

9. Schon D. Educating the Reflective Practitioner: Towards a New Design for Teaching and Learning in the Professions. San Francisco: Jossey Bass; 1987

10. Grol R, Lawrence M. Quality improvement by peer review. New York: Oxford University Press; 1995

CHAPTER 2

SELECT EDUCATIONAL METHODS

FOR REFLECTION

How can you use different educational methods
to achieve your evolving goals over time?

OVERVIEW

As a lifelong learner, you can use learning principles and a variety of educational methods to expand your range and depth of motivational skills. An exercise about learning how to learn will help you explore the merits of using different educational methods to achieve your goals. Both self-directed and collaborative methods are described in detail.

As you develop new skills in role plays and patient encounters, you will experience stuck moments, awkward moments, or "branch points." Bail-out strategies are described to help you handle and learn from these challenging experiences.

SELECT EDUCATIONAL METHODS

Developing motivational skills is more complicated than doing a minor surgical procedure. Yet, in most training programs, little curriculum time is devoted to developing motivational skills. Yet, your nonverbal communication and use of language need the sophistication, precision and grace of a surgeon's hand doing major surgery. Dialogue can help patients cut out their rationalizations and defensive routines that perpetuate their risk behaviors. If successful, patients become less resistant and more receptive to the possibility of change. Furthermore, your words can help patients reflect on, or even change, their values and perceptions so that they become motivated to change. The following exercise may help you select appropriate educational methods for working on your learning goals.

Learning Exercise 2.1: Learning how to Learn[1]
Think about learning two contrasting skills: doing minor surgery and motivating health behavior change. The goal of this exercise is to help you appreciate the importance of practicing a new skill before acting independently, whether it is an interpersonal or a surgical skill. For this exercise, imagine that you have a total of only 40 hours to learn both of these skills. Decide how you would divide the 40 hours for learning these two skills, using Table 2.1.

Table 2.1: Educational Methods for Developing Skills

Options for developing skills	Do minor surgery	Motivate patients
Self-directed Methods		
1. Read about how to do it.		
2. Watch videotapes about how to do it.		
3. Rehearse how to do it.		
4. Assess videotapes of your patient encounters.		
Collaborative Methods		
5. Speak to an experienced clinician about how to do it.		
6. Watch an experienced clinician do it.		
7. Do a rehearsal (simulation/role play).		
8. Review your videotape with a consultant.		
9. Practice with direct supervision.		
10. Practice with patients without supervision.		
11. Consult a colleague when difficulties arise.		
Total hours devoted to learning new skills		

A DEVELOPMENTAL FRAMEWORK

To improve your skills over time, an understanding of learning precepts and different educational methods can help you to develop your learning plan. You can use a skills development framework (Table 2.2) to develop your learning skills along the basic-intermediary-advanced continuum. Using the CPD model as a guide, you can use structured, semi-structured, and unstructured educational methods in self-directed and collaborative ways, but to develop advanced skills, you will need a skilled coach.

Table 2.2: A Skills Development Framework

Developing Basic Skills	Developing Intermediary Skills	Developing Advanced Skills
Self-directed learning	Collaborative learning	Skilled coaches
Well-structured exercises	Semi-structured exercises	Unstructured exercises
Self-focused and method-focused approaches	Learner-centered approaches	Patient-centered approaches

It is important to understand how your work environment can greatly enhance or diminish your prospects of becoming a more effective and efficient motivational practitioner. For this reason, organizational issues are briefly addressed.

ORGANIZATIONAL ISSUES

An organizational perspective provides a larger context in thinking about how to improve the performance of behavior change and disease management programs.[2] Effective organizations work in a population-based manner and support the health care team to adopt motivational roles in working with patients over time. These organizations provide practitioners with ongoing opportunities to enhance their motivational skills and to develop their learning portfolios. In addition, they provide episodic feedback to individual practitioners about the impact of their work on patients, and activate the entire health care team to work on reducing the incidence and prevalence of unhealthy behaviors in their population of patients.

Both educational and clinical data can help the health care team to compile an organizational portfolio that provides evidence about how their CPD programs are improving patient outcomes. Although few organizations currently have such level of support, this situation should not deter them from working toward this long-term goal.

ESSENTIAL LEARNING PRECEPTS

The following precepts can help you enhance your skills at engaging patients in change dialogues over time.

A. Learn how to change yourself before helping others

Your assumptions, roles, perceptions, and values may stand in the way of your becoming an effective motivational practitioner. Knowledge of these issues may help you change, but it may not be sufficient. Effective education helps you become more aware of how personal and professional issues affect your ability to develop skills at motivating behavior change. You will become a more effective health coach if you first learn how to change yourself before helping others.

B. Use self-directed and collaborative educational methods synergistically

Effective use of self-directed and collaborative educational methods can accelerate the development of your motivational skills. Self-directed methods can set up and define how to use your time more productively when using collaborative methods.

C. Find a safe learning environment

A safe, supportive and responsive learning environment helps you use interactive learning methods more effectively to:

- Foster self-reflection, openness, and a willingness to take risks (i.e., avoid being defensive), and share vulnerability.
- Identify, explore, and examine your assumptions, roles, perceptions, attitudes, beliefs, and values.
- Experiment with new ways of thinking, perceiving, and behaving when working with patients (and colleagues).

D. Practice your skills

You become a more effective learner when you actively practice skills rather than passively listen to a lecture about developing skills.[3] Repeated practice sessions can help you enhance your skills and develop new ones. Practice can indeed make "perfect" if the process of reflection and feedback is incorporated into the learning cycle.

E. Reflect about your actions

Reflection is essential for your continuing professional development as a motivational practitioner. There are two kinds of reflection: in the moment (reflection-in-action) and after the event (reflection-on-action). The latter is essential for improving the former.

Reflection-in-action helps you navigate around or through stuck moments, awkward moments, and branch points as they occur in real time. Reflection-on-action refers to your ability to identify, examine and better understand any stuck moments, awkward moments, and branch points that occurred in your role plays or patient encounters after the event. Stuck moments, awkward moments, and branch points should be regarded as gifts for learning something new. Such reflection can help you generate alternative and more effective ways of responding to them when you see the patient the next time or encounter a similar situation. This learning process can in turn expand your repertoire of skills, so that you can reflect more efficiently in the moment during your patient encounters.

F. Work with a mentor

To accelerate your development as a motivational practitioner, you need a trusting relationship with a mentor, facilitator, supervisor, coach or consultant. Such a relationship is essential for soliciting the kind of high-order feedback that will enable you to develop advanced skills more efficiently.

EDUCATIONAL METHODS

You can select any of the following self-directed and/or collaborative educational methods to work on your evolving goals. Because there will never be enough time for using collaborative methods (e.g., small-group learning in CPD programs), it is essential that you develop ways of using self-directed methods on an ongoing basis. Use these methods synergistically with collaborative methods to greatly enhance the quality and impact of your learning experiences.

A. Self-directed Methods

Self-directed methods not only can help you work on many of your learning goals but also clarify how you can use collaborative methods in more effective ways.

1. Address one of your own health behaviors.

Worksheet 1.1a can help you assess your health behaviors and decide whether to change one of them. To work on self-directed change, you can use the MASH guidebook, *Motivate Healthy Habits: Change Yourself Before Helping Others*. This process not only can help you learn how to address your own behavior change, but also can prepare you for using this book with a patient as part of a longitudinal study working with patients over time. These activities can help you better understand professional roles and change concepts to develop new motivational skills more efficiently.

2. Read this two-part practitioner book series.

By studying different theories, models, and interventions, you can expand your knowledge and conceptual understanding about the change process and prepare yourself for developing a new mental map for enhancing your motivational skills over time. Book 1 provides a variety of self-directed learning exercises designed to clarify how you can adopt a motivational role and how you can reflect on assumptions that may help or hinder your work with patients. You will also learn how to apply motivational principles and the six-step approach to patient care.

This book addresses how you can increase your repertoire of skills. For example, Chapters 4b, 5b and 6b use the six-step approach and describe a wide variety of options that you can select to develop individualized interventions for your ambivalent, indifferent, or resistant patients. You can adapt these menus and use your own creativity to initiate dialogues with patients in meaningful and constructive ways.

3. Evaluate video demonstrations of specific tasks and micro skills.

A video demonstration is a helpful way to begin the process of learning how to develop motivational skills. A video at www.MotivateHealthyHabits.com provides an example of how you can use a method-focused approach to complete the three tasks described below:

- Clarify a patient's issues about change (using a decision balance)
- Lower patient resistance (using nondirect interventions)
- Enhance patient motivation (using direct interventions)

Appendix A describes the micro skills for completing these tasks, using tobacco as an example. Watch this Web-based video and then use the checklists in Appendix A to assess your level of understanding in how to use these micro skills, before and after watching this tape. After watching these demonstrations, try and use these micro skills in practice sessions (in role plays or with actual patients) and use the worksheets in Chapter 1 to assess any changes in your level of competence. Before you practice using these skills on actual patients, you need to obtain their consent and inform them that this is a learning opportunity for you.

In following a script, you may feel constrained by this learning process because you may want to follow the patient's lead and address issues outside of the script: in other words, be patient-centered. Method-focused approaches can help you begin to the process of expanding your range and depth of skills, but it can feel unnatural because you are following a script for developing micro skills. If you replicate this demonstration with an actual patient, you are practicing specific skills out of context: in other words, not individualized for that patient.

Such practice sessions, however, do not guarantee that you will be using these micro skills equally well. Learner-centered approaches can help you to improve your overall profile of skills: enhance your strengths and rectify your weaknesses. To shift the focus from yourself to your patients, patient-centered training approaches can help you learn how to develop interventions that meet the patient's changing needs over time.

4. Practice specific tasks and micro skills with a patient.

To assess the impact of using this learning method, you can rate your competence level in using micro skills for the three tasks as demonstrated on the videotape, before and after these practice sessions. You need to ask for your patient's consent to practice (and videotape) doing the three tasks, and then use the one-page handouts in Appendix B. You can say to the patient:

> *"I am learning new ways of helping patients think about changing their behavior* [specify one] *to improve their health. I would like to try a new approach with you. It will take up to an hour. Is that okay? After each practice session, we can both fill out a questionnaire to compare our experiences. In addition, I'd like to ask your opinion about what effect, if any, this approach had on you."*

After completing each task, you and your patient can independently compare perceptions about your interactions, reflect upon your shared experience, and fill out the questionnaires provided in Appendix C. You need to take time out to learn how to use these skills briefly and effectively in routine patient encounters, particularly when you have to deal with time pressures and competing priorities.

In addition, you can adapt this learning and self-assessment process to develop additional micro skills described in the other steps of the six-step approach. Select micro skills from the charts used in Worksheets 1.4-1.9 and create your own one-page guide to use in role plays and patient encounters.

5. Review your own videotapes or audiotapes of patient encounters.

Ask for your patient's consent to videotape your encounter so that you can assess your interactions in a more systematic manner.[4] When engaging in this self-critique, identify first what you did well, and then identify any stuck moments, awkward moments, and/or branch points where you could have responded in alternative and more effective ways. Focusing on the positive aspects of your performance gives you a more balanced perspective on the quality of your encounter with the patient. To gain more from this experience, consider asking the patient to review the tape with you to get additional feedback.

6. Address stuck moments after your practice sessions or in patient encounters.

Reflection-on-action can help you become more adept in addressing stuck moments as they happen. You use the time after a patient encounter to reflect about how to prepare for your next interaction. The example of Mrs. S. used on page 17 in Chapter 1, Book 1 provides an example of getting stuck in working with a patient.

> *Patient Example of Resisting Safe Sex Practices—Mrs. S. (a 45-year-old woman) continued to have unsafe sex with her HIV-positive husband. After establishing that Mrs. S. knew how to put a condom on her husband, MP (motivational practitioner) took a*

different approach. He drew a decision balance and informed Mrs. S. that he would like to better understand why she did not want to use condoms. He asked her if she would be willing to write down her thoughts about the benefits and concerns of unsafe sex and compare them to using condoms every time. To give her privacy, MP left the room and returned about 10 minutes later. Mrs. S. then showed him what she had written.

Mrs. S.'s Decision Balance

Reasons not to use condoms	*Reasons to use condoms*
Benefits of not using condoms *Doesn't make him feel he's sexually incompetent.* *He feels secure that I'll stay with him.*	*Concerns about not using condoms* *Don't want HIV.* *Don't want my family hurt.* *Don't want people to think he doesn't care enough to want to protect me.*
Concerns about using condoms *He will have erection problems, and it will make him sad.* *He will wish he were with his ex-girlfriend (who is HIV positive) so he won't have to use them.*	*Benefits of using condoms* *Won't get HIV so won't upset family.* *Won't get sick myself so I can take care of him when he gets sicker.* *Will feel that he cares enough about me not to allow me to get sick.*

After completing the decision balance, Mrs. S. said that she was willing to sacrifice her life for her husband because she was so in love with him, but she had not shared this information with her husband. The practitioner set up a follow-up appointment and decided to take some time out before the next appointment to think about how best to proceed in working with her.

Learning Exercise 2.2: Developing nondirect interventions

You can use this example of a stuck moment to generate your own list of nondirect interventions to understand better why Mrs. S. did not want to change. Write in an additional example for each of the nondirect interventions.

Use simple reflection: *"So your husband feels sexually incompetent when using a condom?"*

Probe priorities to explore ambivalence: *"So what would be the most important reason for not using condoms?" "And what is the most important reason for using condoms?"*

Use double-sided reflection to summarize ambivalence: *"On the one hand, you want to feel secure with him, but on the other hand, your family will be very upset that you did get HIV by not protecting yourself."*

Acknowledge ambivalence to validate patient's experience: *"You seem to have some mixed feelings about what you are doing because you love your husband so much that you're willing to sacrifice yourself, but you don't want to get HIV either."*

Emphasize personal responsibility and choice (useful when patient is being resistant): *"Only you can decide whether you are willing to use safe sex practice."*

Explore the future to understand the patient's perspectives about her risk behavior: *"If you continue not to use condoms, what do you think your future holds?"*

Learning Exercise 2.3: Developing direct interventions

You can use this example of a stuck moment to generate your own list of direct interventions to help increase Mrs. S.'s motivation to change. Write in an additional example for each of the direct interventions.

Use back-to-the-future questioning: *"What do you think would happen if you contracted HIV and developed AIDS more quickly than your husband so that he had to look after you?"*

Use benefit substitution: *"Are there other ways that you can make your husband feel secure about your staying with him other than by not using condoms?"*

Clarify values: *"What's more important to you—your relationship with your husband or with your family?"*

> Use discrepancies: *"You say that you don't want your family to think that your husband doesn't care to protect you, but they might do so if you get HIV."*

> Reframe issues, items or events: *"Given that you've not contracted HIV for the past 18 months, you may feel that you're especially protected against the virus, but unsafe sex is like a game of Russian roulette."*

> Use differences in motivational reasons: *"Given that you haven't told your family that you're putting yourself at risk, it's clear you're willing to protect the family from this. What would it take for you to protect yourself?"*

This kind of work is very useful for preparing for stuck moment seminars, where you can get additional ideas about how to handle this situation. Don't use an idea unless you feel reasonably comfortable that you are working in your patient's best interest. You may think that you would never say some of the examples provided above to a patient. To help you explore what might work for you and your patient, you can do mini role plays in these seminars to learn whether you can put these ideas into practice.

7. Conduct an in-depth study, working longitudinally with an individual patient.

You can introduce a patient in person to the MASH guidebook by helping him or her fill in a decision balance (described in Chapter 3) to address a particular health behavior. Make a contact (in person, e-mail or via telephone) at a follow-up time convenient to the patient, after the patient has worked on:

- Chapter 3 Get Ready for Change
- Chapter 4 Take Charge of Your Health
- Chapter 5 Make Plans for Change

Ideally, you need repeated contacts with the patient as frequently and for as long as the patient needs it, even if it takes 1-2 years. Though this option is useful for learning purposes but not feasible in clinical practice, its in-depth learning process can better prepare you for clinical practice.

In a similar way that you collected both quantitative and qualitative data from using the MASH guidebook on yourself, you can collect similar data from your patients about the impact of using this guidebook and the additional benefits gained by patients from having episodic contact with you. After each encounter with a patient, you can ask him or her, "What did you find helpful from our conversation today? In what ways could I be more helpful in helping you change?" These questions can clarify the extent to which you were helpful, over and beyond the self-directed change attempts made by your patient in using the guidebook.

B. Collaborative Methods[5]

To help you enhance your range of new skills, you can choose one or more of the following options:

1. Participate in MASH groups to address your health behavior change issue.

In a small group (peer-led or facilitator-led), write out your responses to some learning exercises (downloadable from www.MotivateHealthyHabits.com.) in a three-phase workshop, as outlined below. Each phase can be completed in 40-60 minutes, with 10 to 15 minutes devoted to the writing exercise and 30 to 45 minutes for a discussion responding to the questions listed below. In these small groups, participants are not expected to disclose what health issues they are addressing, but they can share this with the group if they wish. The focus of the group discussions is on learning rather than specific health issues.

- Phase 1—Get Ready for Change (Chapter 3)
  Questions for small-group discussion:
  1. What did you learn from doing this learning exercise that helped you clarify and better understand your issues about change?
  2. What did you learn that was new for you?
  3. How will this new learning help you work with patients?

- Phase 2—Take Charge of Your Health: Lower Your Resistance (Chapter 4a)
  Questions for small-group discussion:
  1. Which learning exercises helped you to lower your resistance scores?
  2. What did you learn that was new for you?
  3. How will this new learning help you work with patients?

- Phase 3—Take Charge of Your Health: Increase Your Motivation (Chapter 4b)
  Questions for small-group discussion:
  1. Which learning exercises helped you to increase your motivation scores?
  2. What did you learn that was new for you?
  3. How will this new learning help you work with patients?

This group work can be done in one session (2-3 hours), but it will be optimal in three or more weekly sessions. After these sessions, you can use Chapter 5 (Make a Plan) from the MASH guidebook to continue working on health behavior change in a self-directed way.

2. Participate in skill development workshops using role plays.

A skill development workshop provides you with opportunities to learn new skills in role plays with colleagues. You may feel reluctant, however, about using this learning method. If so, the following learning exercise may help you explore this issue.

Learning Exercise 2.4: Doing role plays

Practitioners are not allowed to do surgical procedures on patients without appropriate supervision and training. They also need supervised training while learning how to negotiate with patients and motivate behavior change. This exercise can help you to understand the reasons for your reluctance to use this learning method.

Write down in Table 2.3 what you think are the advantages and disadvantages of practicing directly with patients without supervision versus learning how to motivate health behavior change through the use of role plays.

Table 2.3: Reluctance versus Willingness to Use Role Plays

Reluctance to using role plays	*Willingness to use role plays*
Advantages of practicing with patients without supervision	*Disadvantages of practicing with patients without supervision*
Disadvantages of using role plays	*Advantages of using role plays*

If you are more reluctant than willing to participate in role plays, you can develop a better appreciation of your patients' feeling of reluctance. In this instance, you could use your resistance to using this learning method by being a patient in a role play to a colleague who is acting as a practitioner.

Role play guide

A brief guide is provided below on how to conduct role plays, either structured ones that use scripts or self-directed ones that use your own patient examples. These guidelines may allay some concerns about participating in either type of role play. Setup for role plays

- One person plays the "practitioner" role, and the other plays the "patient" role. Each role play lasts 5-8 minutes. (If possible, videotape it.) A detailed guide in Appendix B provides you with one-page handouts for completing these tasks:
  - Clarify a patient's issues about change (using a decision balance)
  - Lower patient resistance (using nondirect interventions)
  - Enhance patient motivation (using direct interventions)

- After each role-playing exercise, the "practitioner" and the "patient" can debrief using checklists in Appendix B, and address the following questions:

For the "practitioner":

- Which interventions worked well on your "patient"?
- How could you improve the interventions you used?

For the "patient":

- Respond to your practitioner's self-critique by sharing your reactions to and thoughts about whether these interventions had a greater or lesser impact than what the practitioner thought or realized.
- Offer suggestions about how the interventions could be used more effectively.

Appendix B provides a comprehensive guide, including handouts, for conducting a three-hour workshop that can be done at one session or three separate hourly sessions. After completing this workshop, you can fill in relevant sections of Worksheets 1.6-1.7 in Chapter 1 to assess any change in your level of competence in developing your micro skills at assessing resistance and motivation and enhancing mutual understanding.

You can also organize role plays based on your experiences of working with your own patients. You can re-enact a particular part of your patient encounter, with your colleague acting as the practitioner. Reenactments are useful when you experience impasses, awkward moments, and branch points during a patient encounter. For example, you can select to practice any of the micro skills described in Chapters 4b, 5b and 6b. Such role plays can help you generate new ways of responding to your patient and allows you to practice being patient-centered in your learning approach. Using the ideas developed from such role plays, you can use your recently acquired skills to address unresolved issues from the previous patient encounter in a follow-up appointment.

Role-playing Exercise—MP (motivational practitioner) decided to do a role play with a colleague who had studied the decision balance. Through the process of conducting this re-enactment, MP discovered a number of different ways to understand why Mrs. S. didn't want to change. He felt it was really important for him to understand more about why Mrs. S. loved her husband so much. MP felt that if Mrs. S. expressed her love openly to her husband and shared her decision balance with him, he might come to appreciate that she has no intention of leaving him.

His colleague mentioned the idea of inviting Mr. S. to the next appointment to find out whether he had a primary care physician, in addition to attending the AIDS clinic. She also suggested that MP consider asking Mrs. S. to ask her husband to fill in a decision balance about using a decision for himself so that they could talk about this further.

Patient Example of Safe Sex Practices—At the next appointment, MP commented on how much Mrs. S. really loved her husband. He then asked her whether her husband was aware of how she was willing to sacrifice her life for him and whether she had told him so. She seemed reluctant to do this. When MP asked Mrs. S. to share the decision balance with her husband, she seemed very receptive to the idea. She also agreed to invite her husband to accompany her to an appointment two weeks after his release from prison to discuss the result of her HIV test.

This kind of work can also be done in stuck moment seminars; see 4. below.

3. Arrange for one-on-one supervision (direct observation or videotape review).

Ask a third party (supervisor, consultant and/or expert) with more advanced skills to directly observe and provide feedback on your patient interaction. Explain the purpose of the encounter to this person and negotiate in advance what sort of feedback you would like directly after the patient encounter.

Alternatively, you can also videotape the patient encounter (with his or her consent) for a more in-depth review with your supervisor. Review your videotape before the session to identify impasses or missed opportunities in working with your patient, and generate your own ideas about how you could have handled these situations better. Share your ideas with this person before asking for additional ideas.

4. Organize small-group seminars for stuck moments and longitudinal case studies.

Identify your stuck moments with patients. Make notes about them. Better still, tape record or videotape patient encounters so that you can capture brief vignettes of your stuck moments with patients. You can use your stuck moment examples in these seminars.

a. Stuck Moment Seminars

A suggested plan for conducting small-group seminars (30-60 minutes) on stuck moments is outlined below.

Preparation for role play
1. With ongoing small groups, presenters from previous sessions give updates about their patients.
2. Participants generate a list of stuck moments from patient encounters.
3. Participants vote on which patient to discuss.
4. A presenter provides background information and describes the stuck moment.
5. The presenter provides ideas on how to improve this situation.
6. A scribe makes a note of these ideas on a flipchart or blackboard.
7. The group brainstorms about additional ideas for handling the situation.
8. The scribe also notes the name of the person who provides the additional ideas.
9. The presenter rank orders the merit of these ideas for the practice session.

Role plays
1. The presenter plays the role of the patient.
2. The identified person enacts his or her idea in a mini role play (2-5 minutes).
3. The "practitioner" notes what worked well and then generates additional ideas about how to improve what was done.
4. The presenter "patient" notes what the practitioner did well, and then generates additional ideas on improving what was done.
5. The group provides additional feedback about the interaction and additional ideas about handling the stuck moment.
6. The presenter selects the next idea and repeats steps 1-5.

Debriefing role plays
1. The presenter identifies what he or she will do differently with the patient.
2. The group shares what they learned that was new for them.
3. The presenter uses the notes from the session to keep a journal about the patient interactions over time.
4. The presenter for the next session is identified.

You can also address stuck moments in consultation with other experienced clinicians or experts, either in person, or in consultations via e-mail.

b. Longitudinal Case Studies

You can use the MASH guidebook with a patient. Introduce the guidebook to a patient in person and help him or her select an unhealthy behavior and fill in a decision balance, as described in Chapter 3 of that guide. Make a minimum of three follow-up contacts (in person, e-mail or on the telephone) at a pace convenient to the patient, after the patient has worked on:

- Chapter 3 Get Ready for Change
- Chapter 4 Take Charge of Your Health
- Chapter 5 Make a Plan

Ideally, you need repeated contacts with the patient as frequently and for as long as the patient needs it, even if it takes 1-2 years.

In a similar way that you collected qualitative data from using this guidebook on yourself, you can collect similar data from the patients about the impact of using this MASH guidebook and the additional benefits gained by patients from having episodic contact with you. After each encounter with a patient, you can ask him or her, "What did you find helpful from our conversation today? In what ways could I be more helpful in helping you change?"

5. Use mentors and reflection groups to address personal and professional issues.
Even when you use effective training methods, you may still encounter difficulties in particular situations that relate to your own personal and professional issues. You will learn how to work more effectively with these situations if you use mentors or consultee-focused groups to address issues that hinder your ability to work as a motivational practitioner.

a. Mentors
You can consult a more experienced practitioner to act as a mentor to help you work through your particular issues. The following example provides a specific issue of how a personal issue affects professional work, and it also shows the benefits of direct observation.

A mentor was watching a trainee working with a pregnant teenager who had high-risk sexual behaviors. The teenager was reluctant to have an HIV test. The mentor and trainee stepped out of the room to discuss how to address this issue. The mentor suggested using a decision balance with the teenager and gave specific instructions about how to initiate this task in 60 seconds. Even though the trainee had experience in this technique, he had difficulties in providing this teenager with a rationale for using a decision balance. He used too many words and avoided being direct with the teenager. The teenager sensed his difficulties. The trainee became embarrassed, sensing that the teenager perceived his difficulties in initiating this task. Nonetheless, the teenager cooperated and agreed to think about having the test. Afterwards, the mentor complemented the trainee on his sensitive style and his ability in being nondirect with this teenager and allowing her to express openly her preference about not getting HIV tested. The mentor asked the trainee if he were willing to share his perspective about his difficulties in completing this task. He disclosed that he was unsuccessful in persuading his current girlfriend to get HIV-tested. The mentor asked the trainee if he had difficulties being direct with people in general, or just in dealing with sexual issues. The trainee had had difficulties in being direct with people, and disliked dealing with conflicts for fear of upsetting others. The mentor suggested that it may help to have some additional coaching sessions to handle this situation more effectively and/or to explore these personal issues with a counselor. The trainee chose the coaching sessions but was willing to consider a counselor if this approach did not work.

b. Reflection Groups

Balint groups, Family Systems Balint groups, personal awareness groups, and reflection groups may enhance your self-awareness and, as a result, your effectiveness as a facilitator in these difficult situations.[6-10] A variety of methods can be used to address the personal and professional issues that affect your ability to work with indifferent, ambivalent, and resistant patients. These include exploring transference and countertransference issues and addressing family-of-origin issues relevant to both the patient and yourself: in other words, what are the issues you and your patients bring to your interaction that you project on one another and that interfere with how well you can work together?

Reflection groups help practitioners understand what it is about themselves that make it particularly difficult to work with certain patients. The following example shows how a practitioner used a reflection group to help her address a challenging experience in which a personal issue was affecting her performance.

Moira Dickinson is a 48-year-old nurse practitioner whose father died at the age of 52 from a heart attack due to a variety of cardiovascular risk factors: diabetes, smoking, obesity, and high cholesterol. She found it particularly frustrating to work with diabetic male patients with similar risk factors. One of the patients she worked with, Mr. G. (55 years old), always seemed to be doing well when discussing health issues during office visits, but his blood sugar levels were invariably elevated. In spite of diligently instructing him on the use of a sliding scale for varying meal sizes, Moira heard from Mrs. G. that Mr. G. did not adhere to the diet stringently, nor did he adjust his insulin according to meal size. Mrs. G. also mentioned that Mr. G. had informed her that he was thinking about seeing a doctor for his condition. His wife did not think this was necessary because she thought Moira was doing a good job.

Moira felt particularly frustrated because she desperately wanted to help Mr. G. avoid having a heart attack. Unknown to her, however, Mr. G. felt that she was nagging him too much. In spite of being well trained in the use of negotiation strategies and motivational interventions, she had forthrightly advised Mr. G. to control his diabetes better and reduce his cardiovascular risk factors. In this case, Moira was more invested in change than he was. Given the difficulties in working with Mr. G., Moira decided to discuss this patient with colleagues in a reflection group because she recognized that the harder she tried to help Mr. G. change, the less he seemed motivated to do so.

In Moira's own family, she identified with her mother, who had tried to persuade her father not to overeat. Moira felt particularly guilty and angry at herself that, while a nurse in training, she had not helped her mother more in trying to get her father to quit smoking and take better care of his diabetes, high cholesterol, and obesity. In discussing these issues with colleagues, Moira began to realize that she was taking too much responsibility for Mr. G. and was not giving him the opportunity to decide whether, when, and how to modify his cardiovascular risk factors. As a result of the group discussion and further self-reflection, Moira felt less need to pressure Mr. G. and instead thought of new ways to help him choose which risk factors to work on first. She negotiated with Mr. G about setting some realistic goals rather than trying to address everything at once. Although she already knew how to do this, her emotional buttons had been pushed with Mr. G and so she felt an overwhelming need to make him change.

Moira later shared with the reflection group that Mr. G. subsequently attended appointments with his ophthalmologist on a regular basis, that his wife organized his meals more in accordance with the recommended diet, that he kept a better record of his blood sugar levels, and that he inspected his feet on a regular basis. In turn, Moira began to make a more balanced assessment of both the negative and positive aspects of Mr. G.'s behaviors. Positive outcomes included a slight improvement in his blood glucose and a 5-pound weight loss.

If you want to learn more about the small group process, use of videotapes, and role plays, you can refer to these referenced texts.[3;4;4;11-21]

6. Review individual and group performance at team meetings.

In ideal health care settings, practitioners are given regular reports about their individual and group performance in terms of reducing the incidence and prevalence of unhealthy behaviors among their panel of patients. This can help practitioners determine whether their learning plan is having an impact on patients and how their soft (psychosocial) data gathered in their learning portfolio relates to these hard outcomes—in other words, how the process of their continuing professional development plans helps to improve both their competence and performance in working with patients over time. Alternatively, you can gather a series of case reports to report the impact of your work.

BAIL-OUT STRATEGIES

You can use any of the bail-out strategies described below to overcome impasses and awkward moments that are bound to happen sometimes when practicing new skills. You take a risk whenever you use a new skill with a patient. If you feel particularly uncomfortable about using a technique, try to understand why you feel reluctant about using it, and identify a specific bail-out strategy that you can use in the event that the technique does not work for you. In other words, don't jump without a parachute.

1. Check whether an intervention is working.

When using new interventions, you may have difficulty knowing what effect they have on a patient. Sometimes, you will be surprised. Check it out with your patients, because you may find you are doing a better job than you thought.

Suggested language:
"I just tried a new approach for helping people think about change. I'd like to know whether or not you found it helpful. What do you think?"

2. Clarify the source of awkwardness.

When practicing using any new skill, you may initially feel awkward because it does not fit in with your normal pattern of interacting with patients. Patients may sense your awkwardness but still feel that the interaction itself was effective. Sometimes awkwardness arises from the practitioner-patient interaction itself; at other times, you yourself may not feel awkward using a new skill but may still make the patient feel awkward. You may even find it difficult to know where the sense or feeling of awkwardness is coming from. Addressing and clarifying the source of your awkward or uncomfortable feelings can help you better understand the challenge of change for the patient as well as for yourself.

Suggested language:
"I felt awkward when I said_____. Did it affect you in any way?"
"When I said_____, it felt awkward between us. How did it feel to you?"
"When I said_____, I felt that it made you feel awkward. [Let patient respond and, if prompting is necessary, proceed further.] *Can you help me understand that?"*

Remember that these options are to create opportunities for you and your patients to learn from your interactions in ways that will facilitate change.

3. Comment on the process.

You can comment on the process of what is happening or not happening in the interaction, rather than pushing to work on what you think the patient needs to address.

Suggested language:
"I sense that we're not working on the same wavelength."
"I sense that we're working at cross purposes."
"I get the sense that you don't think that I'm trying to work on your side."
"A moment ago, I tried to help you increase your motivation to change, but it isn't clear to me whether or not you want me to help you."

4. Take a timeout.

On rare occasions when none of these bail-out strategies seem to work for you, you can tell patients that you need to take a timeout.

Suggested language:
"I get a sense that what we're trying to do is just not working. I'm wondering whether we should drop this for now so that we can think more about it and come back to it later. What do you think?"

5. Consult others.

When you get stuck, reach an impasse, or are uncertain about what to do about a health care issue, you can consult your colleagues or encourage patients to consult family members and friends. This strategy sends your patient the message that more time and attention is needed to address the issue.

> *Suggested language:*
> *"I'm not quite sure how to proceed from this point. I think it's very important that we address this issue more, but I would like to speak to a colleague first to think through how you and I can work together more effectively."*
> *"I think this issue is particularly important for you, but I think it might be worthwhile for you to talk to your family members and friends to find out what they think about this issue. Afterward, we can get back together and talk about it more."*

MOVING ON

The synergistic use of self-directed and collaborative educational methods can accelerate your development as a motivational practitioner. You need to select, however, which methods can best help you achieve your learning goals. The next chapter describes how you can create and organize a learning portfolio. A learning portfolio provides you with an opportunity to provide evidence that demonstrates what you have learned, how you have changed, what you can do differently, and how this can benefit others.

Reference List

1. Jason H, Westberg J. You as a learner. Medical Teachers 1981;3: 73-75
2. Skinner HA. Promoting Health through Organizational Change. San Francisco: Benjamin Cummings; 2002
3. Knowles M. The adult learner: A neglected species. Fourth ed. Houston, TX: Gulf Publishing Co.; 1990
4. Westberg J, Jason H. Teaching creatively with video. New York, NY: Springer Publishing Co.; 1994
5. Westberg J, Jason H. Collaborative education: Preparing health professionals for functioning as partners. 1995:1-17
6. Balint M. The doctor, his patient, and the illness. New York: International Universities Press; 1977
7. Brock C. Balint group leadership by a family physician in a residency program. Family Medicine 1985;17: 61-63
8. Samuel O. How doctors learn in a Balint group. Family Practice 1989;6: 108-113
9. Schemgold L. Balint work in England: Lessons for American Family Medicine. Journal of Family Practice 1988;26: 315-320
10. Botelho RJ, McDaniel SH, Jones JE. A family systems approach to a Balint-style group: A report on a CME demonstration project for primary care physicians. Family Medicine 1990;22: 293-295

11. Westberg J, Jason H. Fostering learning in small groups: A practical guide. New York, NY: Springer Publishing Company, Inc.; 1996

12. Fabb WE, Heffernan MW, Phillips WA, et al. Focus on learning in family practice. Melbourne, Australia: Royal Australian College of General Practitioners; 1976

13. Westberg J, Jason H. Providing constructive feedback. Boulder, CO: The Center for Instructional Support; 1991

14. Bruffee KA. Collaborative learning: Higher education, interdependence, and the authority of knowledge. Baltimore, MD: The Johns Hopkins University Press; 1993

15. Vella J. Training through dialogue: Promoting effective learning and change with adults. San Francisco, CA: Jossey-Bass Inc.; 1995

16. Havelock P, Hasler J, Flew R, et al. Professional education for general practice. New York: Oxford University Press; 1995

17. Horder J, Byrne P, Freeling P, et al. The future general practitioner: Learning and teaching. London: The British Medical Journal; 1972

18. Farquharson A. Teaching in practice. San Francisco, CA: Jossey-Bass; 1995

19. Douglas KC, Hosokawa MC, Lawler FH. A practical guide to clinical teaching in medicine. New York: Springer Publishing Co., Inc.; 1988

20. Cormack J, Marinker M, Morrell D. Teaching general practice. London: Kluwer Publishing Ltd.; 1981

21. vanMents M. The effective use of role play: A handbook for teachers & trainers. Revised ed. New York: Nichols Publishing; 1989

CHAPTER 3
CREATE A LEARNING PORTFOLIO

FOR REFLECTION

How can you create a learning portfolio that demonstrates how the process of your continuing professional development improves patient care outcomes?

OVERVIEW

A learning portfolio is a carefully compiled collection of evidence that demonstrates how different educational methods helped to enhance your:

- Ability to change your own health behaviors and to adopt a motivational role
- Understanding about motivational principles and the six-step approach
- Competence, capabilities and skills
- Performance (improved patient care outcomes)

The process of creating a learning portfolio can help you maintain your enthusiasm and curiosity about learning from your experiences in how to motivate patients to change over time. This process is driven by the need to improve patient care outcomes. A learning portfolio not only reinforces what you have learned but also helps you gather evidence about the process of your continuing professional development. You can gather a spectrum of evidence across the four phases of the CPD model: self-focused, method-focused, learner-centered and patient-centered.

CREATE A LEARNING PORTFOLIO

CLARIFYING THE PURPOSE

The ultimate goal in creating a learning portfolio for developing motivational skills is to enhance the effectiveness of behavior change and disease management programs by improving health care outcomes at a population-based level. This long-term goal involves a series of intermediary developmental objectives. A learning portfolio can help you gather a spectrum of evidence that demonstrates how different educational methods helped to enhance your ability to change your own health behaviors and to adopt a motivational role, and your understanding, skills, competence, capabilities, and performance.[1-3] It is important to understand the distinction between competence and capabilities. Capability is more than competence.[4]

- Competence—what individuals know or are able to do in terms of knowledge, understanding, skills, and attitudes.

- Capability—extent to which individuals can adapt to change, generate new knowledge, and continue to improve performance.

Your learning portfolio can present a spectrum of evidence across the four phases of the CPD model.

- Self-focused—documents how you have changed your own health behavior, enhanced your understanding about differences between the fix-it and motivational roles, and increased your competence in adopting a motivational role.

- Method-focused—documents how you have enhanced your understanding about motivational principles and specific micro skills in the six-step approach before and after watching a video demonstration.

- Learner-centered—documents how you have enhanced your range and depth of motivational skills.

- Patient-centered—documents how you have developed individualized interventions for patients, reduced the rate of risk behaviors, and improved patient care outcomes over time.

ORGANIZING YOUR PORTFOLIO

Your learning goals are the starting point in creating your learning portfolio. Key components include: conducting self-assessments; clarifying educational needs; setting objectives; selecting educational methods; identifying, selecting and using resources; reflecting about learning experiences; soliciting feedback from peers, mentors and supervisors; gathering different kinds of qualitative and quantitative evidence about your progress on achieving your goals; and making suggestions for improvement.

There are many ways to organize a learning portfolio. Rather than impose a particular structure, you can create your own way of incorporating these key components to accommodate your learning experiences and style. Your portfolio can be informal (purely for your own benefit), or formal (used as part of an evaluation process). Here are some suggestions about how to organize a formal portfolio.

- Title page with learner's name, year of training, and name of mentor.
- List of learning objectives and timetable.
- Episodic progress reports under each learning objective. Describe how your educational methods helped you achieve your goals by providing different kinds of evidence: episodic self-assessments;[5-7] reflection notes about reading articles, chapters, books, and small group learning experiences; critical learning events and reviews;[8] accounts of overcoming "stuck" moments with patients; formal presentations; peer or patient testimonials or feedback;[9] evaluation of videotaped patient encounters;[10] semi-structured interview of patients; and narrative analysis of practitioner-patient transcripts. [11]
- Record of episodic reviews of your learning portfolio with your mentor.
- Summary statements for review with your mentor

The worksheets in Chapter 1 provide the foundation for developing your learning goals. In addition, you can use the PARE improvement cycle to gather evidence for your learning portfolio to document your continuing professional development: change yourself personally and professionally; deepen your knowledge and understanding about behavior change; enhance your competence by expanding your repertoire of motivational skills; enhance your capabilities; and improve patient outcomes. Using this improvement cycle as a guide, your learning plan will consist of four sections:

- **Prepare**—Photocopy the worksheets. Conduct self-assessments, rate your understanding and competence in addressing behavior change, develop your learning goals, and set a timetable for working on your goals.
- **Act**—Select educational methods (see Chapter 2) to achieve your goals. Document the methods you used.
- **Reflect**—Assess the impact of your educational methods on achieving your

goals by using the worksheets to rate yourself again. Write down your reasons for any change in your scores and provide additional data to justify the changes in your scores (third-party opinion, videotapes, improved patient outcomes). Gather additional evidence (such as videotapes of simulated or actual patient encounters) for your learning portfolio.

- **Enhance**—Use this learning experience to refine your learning goals so that you can work through the PARE cycle again.

CONDUCTING ASSESSMENTS

Colleagues and mentors can provide assessments on your progress on achieving your goals and feedback on how to improve your learning portfolio. Such meetings can be formal or informal, scheduled or unscheduled. These exchanges can be in person, or via the telephone, the Web or the Internet.

Both summative and formative assessments, conducted by you and by third parties (patients, peers, supervisors, and expert consultant) can help you gather evidence for your learning portfolio. It is important to understand the distinctions between these assessments before moving ahead.

Summative assessments are tests that grade your knowledge, skills and/or performance level at specific times during your training. These tests are important for ensuring that you have reached a predetermined benchmark or standard; however, they do not adequately measure how much you have learned and what you want to learn in the future. With formative assessments, third parties (teachers, peers and colleagues) give you feedback about how you are doing and how to improve. These single or episodic events can be planned or opportunistic. Such assessments are essential for improving your competence and performance during training; for this reason, they are more helpful than summative assessments for enhancing your competence and performance.

After completing your training period, self-assessment skills are even more essential for your continuing professional development. Such assessments help you understand better where you were, where you are now, and where you want to go: in other words, how much more you can improve. Self-assessment skills, however, are difficult to acquire in time-pressured, competitive atmospheres of professional training programs that predominantly rely on summative assessments and provide little time for formative assessments. Such programs can create a low-trust educational atmosphere that can create significant barriers to lifelong learning. These programs can make you feel reluctant about conducting self-assessments and reviewing videotapes (or audiotapes) of your practice sessions or patient encounters. Furthermore, they may not even provide you with opportunities for learning about how to develop your self-assessment skills during your formal education.

GATHERING EVIDENCE

The four phases of the CPD model (self-focused, method-focused, learner-centered, and patient-centered) provide an overall framework to gather a spectrum of evidence. The following descriptions of each phase have a purposeful, repetitive format. Practice and repetition that focuses on your specific educational needs is an essential learning process for skills development. Real examples of learning plans are downloadable from the Web site www.MotivateHealthyHabits.com. This will give you a much better feel for how you can actually design your individualized learning plan and organize your learning portfolio.

A. Self-focused Evidence
1. Document changes in your health behaviors.

Worksheet 1.1a can help you pick a health behavior to improve. To gather evidence about changes in your health behaviors, the MASH guidebook provides a variety of learning exercises to help you get ready for change (Chapter 3), take charge of your health (Chapter 4), and make plans for change (Chapter 5). As you work through the exercises in these chapters, you can use the SEED improvement cycle repeatedly over time to make your progress toward your goals. This cycle consists of four steps:

- Study—select an exercise to read
- Exercise—write out a response to the exercise
- Evaluate—assess the helpfulness of the exercise
- Document—use the progress charts to monitor progress toward your goals

Appendix A in the MASH guidebook provides a progress chart for monitoring changes in your scores for:

- Resistance and motivation based on how you think and feel
- Level of energy and priorities devoted toward change
- Motives for change
- Confidence and ability to change

Such documentation provides evidence for your learning portfolio.

In addition to this self-directed learning, you can use the MASH guidebook in small groups. For example, you can discuss which learning exercises helped you change, so that you can learn more from one another. You can then document how small-group learning helped you learn more about motivating behavior change, beyond your work on self-directed change.

2. Document your enhanced understanding about professional roles.
Prepare: Make notes about the reasons for your scores in the checklist in Worksheet 1.1b.
Act: Read Chapters 2 and 3 in Book 1.
Reflect: Use the checklist in Worksheet 1.1b to score these items again. Make notes about the reasons for changing your scores.
Enhance: Suggest ideas for improvement based on your learning experience. Refine your goals. Repeat the PARE improvement cycle, with or without using the worksheet.

These notes provide qualitative data about how you have enhanced your understanding about professional roles and increase your competence to act as a motivational practitioner over time. Such data can provide insights in how you are enhancing your depth and level of understanding about professional roles.

B. Method-focused Evidence
1. Document your enhanced understanding of motivational principles.
Prepare: Make notes about the reasons for your baseline scores in Worksheet 1.2a.
Act: Read Book 1.
Reflect: Use Worksheet 1.2a to score these items again. Make notes about the reasons for changing your scores.
Enhance: Suggest ideas for improvement based on your learning experience. Refine your goals. Repeat the PARE improvement cycle, with or without using the worksheet.

2. Document your enhanced understanding about the six-step approach.
Prepare: Make notes about the reasons for your baseline scores in Worksheet 1.2b.
Act: Read Chapter 8 (and for more details Chapters 9-14) in Book 1.
Reflect: Use Worksheet 1.2b to score these items again. Make notes about the reasons for changing your scores. Book 1 also encourages you to make notes after completing Chapters 9-14. These notes can become part of your learning portfolio.
Enhance: Suggest ideas for improvement based on your learning experience. Refine your goals. Repeat the PARE improvement cycle, with or without using the worksheet.

C. Learner-centered Evidence
1. Document how you have improved the way you address different health behaviors.
Use Worksheet 1.3 to makes notes about the reasons you gave yourself your baseline scores, and develop your learning goals based on this self-assessment. Make notes about the reasons for any changes in your scores after reading the books and after you have had some practice sessions.

Prepare: Make notes about the reasons for your baseline scores in Worksheet 1.3.
Act: Work on improving your ability to address your different health behaviors.
Reflect: Use Worksheet 1.3 to score these items again. Make notes about the reasons for changing your scores.
Enhance: Suggest ideas for improvement based on your learning experience. Refine your goals. Repeat the PARE improvement cycle, with or without using the worksheet.

2. Document how you have improved your micro skills.

You can choose to work on any category of micro skills in the six-step approach.
Prepare: Make notes about the reasons for your baseline scores in Worksheets 1.4-1.9, before or after reading a chapter.
Act: Read the corresponding chapter (9-14) in Book 1 or the relevant sections in Chapter 4b, 5b, or 6b in this book. Practice specific micro skills in role plays.
Reflect: Use the appropriate worksheet to score these items again. Make notes about the reasons for changing your scores.
Enhance: Suggest ideas for improvement based on your learning experience. Refine your goals. Repeat the PARE improvement cycle, with or without using the worksheet.

D. Patient-centered Evidence

Conducting self-assessments on the process of developing motivational skills is challenging because your dialogue with patients is a dynamic and complex process. It can be difficult to do and also reflect about how you are doing during such encounters. Videotaped or audiotaped reviews can help you reflect on these interactional processes after the clinical encounter has occurred; in other words, you keep the "A" (Act) and the "R" (Reflect) separate in using the PARE improvement cycle. This process can help you:

- Identify what you did well but did not recognize during your interaction
- Identify stuck moments, awkward moments, and branch points
- Identify areas for improvement

After your patient encounter, you can ask the patient specific questions about what happened at particular moments.

1. Document how you have improved your ability to address stuck moments.
Prepare: Make notes about your challenges or stuck moments in trying to work in a patient-centered manner. Select educational methods for addressing your challenges or stuck moments with patients.
Act: Implement your educational plan.
Reflect: Make notes about what you learned to help your patient.
Enhance: Develop ideas and use them in your work with patients.
Repeat the cycle until you have successfully worked through your clinical challenges or overcome your stuck moments.

2. Document how you helped a patient change over time.
To gather evidence about how you have helped your patients change over time, you can use the MASH guidebook with a patient and arrange at least three follow-up contacts (in person, via e-mail, or on the telephone), after the patient has completed Chapters 3-5. You can gather data about how the patient used the guidebook in a self-directed way, and how you provided additional help to the patient in addressing behavior change. This process will help you understand better how a patient can address change in a self-directed way and how you can give help and support to the patient.

3. Document reduction in the rates of unhealthy behaviors among your patients.
Prepare: Attend quarterly team meetings to review individual and group performance in terms of reducing the incidence and prevalence of unhealthy behaviors among the panel of patients.
Action: Implement a plan for improving both individual and/or organizational improvement.
Reflect: Assess the impact of the impact on the organization, practitioners and/or patients (for example, how soft data gathered in their learning portfolios relate to hard patient outcomes).
Enhance: Develop ideas and use them to prepare for the next improvement cycle.

MOVING ON

This chapter describes how you can use the four phases of the CPD model and the PARE improvement cycles to create a learning portfolio, documenting how personal and professional changes improved your competence, capabilities, performance and patient care outcomes. The next section presents specific issues relevant to developing micro skills to address three particular risk behaviors: smoking, excessive alcohol use, and self-care of diabetes.

Reference List

1. Challis MC. Personal Learning Plans. Medical Teacher 2000;22: 225-236

2. Mathers NJ, Challis MC, Howe AC, et al. Portfolios in continuing medical education—effective and efficient? [see comments]. Med Educ 1999;33: 521-530

3. Challis MC. Portfolio based learning and assessment in medical education. (AMEE Medical Education Guide No. 11 (revised). Medical Teacher 1999;221: 370-386

4. Fraser SW, Greenhalgh T. Coping with complexity: educating for capability. BMJ 2001;323: 799-803

5. Gordon MJ. Cutting the Gordian knot: a two-part approach to the evaluation and professional development of residents. Acad Med 1997;72: 876-880

6. Gordon MJ. Self-assessment programs and their implications for health professions training. Acad Med 1992;67: 672-679

7. Gordon MJ. A review of the validity and accuracy of self-assessments in health professions training. Acad Med 1991;66: 762-769

8. Flanagan JC. The critical incident technique. Psychological Bulletin 1954;51(4): 327-358

9. Westberg J, Jason H. Fostering Reflection and Providing Feedback. New York City: Springer Publishing Co.; 2001

10. Westberg J, Jason H. Teaching creatively with video. New York, NY: Springer Publishing Co.; 1994

11. Greenhalgh T, Hurwitz B. Narrative Based Medicine: Dialogue and Discourse in Clinical Practice. London: BMJ Books; 1998

SECTION II

SPECIFIC BEHAVIORS

Chapters 4, 5 and 6 address the subject of excessive use of alcohol, smoking, and self-care of diabetes respectively. Each chapter is broken down into two parts; the first part discusses facts and issues specific to the particular behavior, while the second part provides options for developing learning skills based on the six-step model described in Book 1. Each chapter also reinforces how you can adapt this six-step approach to address other risk behaviors. Whatever your time limit in clinical encounters and the number of individual contacts, you can select from the options described to help motivate patients to change their risk behaviors.

A. KEY FINDINGS AND SPECIFIC ISSUES

Chapter 4a describes the notion of a risk continuum, the concept of harm reduction, and the use of uncertainty to assess alcohol problems. Any reduction in risk and harm is worthwhile, particularly when patients cannot attain the ideal goal of total alcohol abstinence. This problem is also relevant to other risk behaviors such as dietary adherence and weight reduction.

Chapter 5a addresses the need to integrate behavioral interventions with drug treatment of nicotine dependence in order to decrease smoking rates. Combining behavioral counseling with medical treatments is also relevant to helping patients overcome other drug addictions.

Chapter 6a addresses self-care of diabetes and the need for patients to juggle multiple agendas. This issue is also applicable to other patients who have multiple risk factors, whether or not they have a chronic disease.

B. DEVELOPING SKILLS

Chapters 4b, 5b, and 6b use the six-step approach, and offer a range of options in each step to help you select the most appropriate interventions for an individual patient at a particular moment in time. These options provide a wealth of ideas, and encourage you to use your clinical judgment in selecting interventions that will enhance your patients' readiness to change.

If you provide continuity of care to patients, you will have multiple opportunities to intervene over time and to develop your professional skills. Your individualized approach can help patients:

- Think more about change
- Reduce their resistance to change
- Enhance their motivation to change
- Prepare for change
- Take action to change

Some options are used more than others. For example, you may use the decision balance more frequently than explicitly clarifying your roles with your patients. The important point is to select and use whatever options seem to work for your individual patient.

CHAPTER 4a

EXCESSIVE ALCOHOL USE

FOR REFLECTION

What is the alcohol risk-and-harm continuum?
How can you use diagnostic uncertainty to assess for alcohol abuse and dependency?

OVERVIEW

Brief interventions have been proven to have a positive effect on excessive alcohol intake. To understand the patterns of alcohol use, an alcohol risk-and-harm continuum lists them in descending order of severity, from alcohol dependence to abstinence. Both alcohol abuse and dependency can be classified from mild to moderate to severe. Definitions for each of these terms are provided in this chapter to assist you and your patients when negotiating about a diagnosis. When you are unable to make such a diagnosis, this chapter discusses how you can use diagnostic uncertainty to help patients assess their excessive use of alcohol.

EXCESSIVE ALCOHOL USE

KEY FACTS

Excessive alcohol use causes massive negative effects on society in health, social and economic consequences.[1;2] Primary care provides multiple opportunities for intervention,[3-9] and mounting evidence supports educating practitioners about using brief interventions with patients who have excessive alcohol intake. [10-14] The overall effect of brief interventions is estimated to be a 24% reduction in alcohol consumption (95% confidence interval, 18%-31%).[10] Yet, many practitioners remain unconvinced or skeptical about the benefits of these interventions.[15;16]

The majority of randomized studies have shown that patients receiving brief interventions have better outcomes than those in control groups with respect to: reducing alcohol consumption, gamma glutamyl-transferase levels, absenteeism from work, alcohol-related problems, hospitalization days, and/or mortality for excessive drinkers in hospital and primary care settings.[17-19;20-32] In a primary care study conducted by Wallace and colleagues, the study group that was given brief advice by general practitioners reported a 17.8% greater reduction in alcohol consumption compared with the control group.[23]

The results of this landmark British study were replicated in a U.S. study.[33] At the time of the 12-month follow-up, significant reductions were achieved in the intervention group, which received brief advice about reducing alcohol consumption, compared to routine care in the control group. The mean number of drinks in the previous weeks decreased from 19.1 to 11.5 for the intervention group vs. 18.9 to 15.5 drinks per week for the control group. The control group had about a 20% reduction in their alcohol use, a finding that was similar to the Wallace et al. study.[23] This raises the issue of whether these changes came about because the control group members were encouraged by participating in lifestyle assessments, or whether the changes represent a regression to the mean.

Another significant finding is that binge drinking was reduced in the intervention group from 5.7 to 3.1 episodes per month after one year, vs. 5.3 to 4.2 episodes per month after 12 months for the control group. (Binge drinking for women is defined as having more than four drinks on one occasion; for men, more than five drinks on one occasion.) Overall, physician advice reduced the alcohol consumption of patients by four drinks per week, and binge drinking by 1.5 episodes per month.

Men and women in the experimental group had a 14% and 31% reduction in alcohol consumption, respectively. With respect to health care utilizations, there was no difference in the number of emergency department visits between the experimental and control groups for either men or women. Men in the control group, however, experienced significantly more self-reported days in hospitals than those in the experimental group: 314 days vs. 178 days. No difference was reported in the number of self-reported hospital days between the two groups for women. This raises the question of why a lower reduction in overall alcohol consumption resulted in fewer hospitalization days for men, but not for women. One possible answer is that in this study, the average age was much higher for men than for women, indicating that age may certainly be a contributing factor.

It is important to note that the British and U.S. studies had different definitions of what is considered to be low-risk drinking. Furthermore, practitioners vary in what they regard as safe, low-risk social drinking.[34] For this reason, national advisory bodies have attempted to define what constitutes low-risk drinking. This issue has been and remains a source of debate. Controversy exists in terms of defining the cutoff for low-risk drinking limits because moderate amounts of alcohol (less than three drinks per day) are also associated with enhanced longevity, reduced cardiovascular mortality, and reduced ischemic (but not hemorrhagic) stroke rate.[35-40] It is difficult to determine epidemiologically exactly where a significant increase in risk begins. As a consequence, countries vary in how they define low-risk drinking.[35]

Furthermore, these research studies excluded patients who were dependent on alcohol. Another challenge of applying the results of these studies to practice becomes how to deal with patients who, unknown to you, are dependent on alcohol.

SPECIFIC ISSUES

When addressing the subject of excessive alcohol use, a number of issues need to be examined to better understand patterns of alcohol use, the risks and harms of such use, and the challenges you face when trying to make a diagnosis.

A. Alcohol Risk-and-harm Continuum

The alcohol risk-and-harm continuum (the patterns of alcohol use) consists of abstinence, low-risk use, hazardous use, harmful (abuse) use of alcohol, and alcohol dependence, each of which, excluding abstinence, will be discussed below. The percentage of the population that suffers from alcohol abuse and dependence is approximately 15%-20% and 5%, respectively. The percentage of the population that uses alcohol hazardously varies from country to country depending on the definition of low-risk drinking and the abstinence rate. The patient's pattern of alcohol use itself can also change over time.

An important issue to consider is what level of prevention (primary, secondary or tertiary) would have the greatest impact on improving the health of the population. Although the health and economic impact of harmful and hazardous drinking (secondary prevention) greatly exceeds that resulting from alcohol dependency,[41] far greater resources are expended on treating alcohol dependency (tertiary prevention in specialist treatment facilities) than in addressing the harmful and hazardous use of alcohol (secondary prevention in primary care and hospital settings). This is despite the fact that secondary prevention approaches have a far greater potential for improving the health of the population at large than tertiary prevention.[42;43] In the U.S. general population, the implementation of safe drinking limits (secondary prevention) would result in an estimated 14.2% and 47.1% reduction in the prevalence of alcohol abuse and dependency, respectively.[44] To reverse the "prevention paradox," health care organizations must systematically introduce secondary prevention programs into mainstream practice. [45;46 47;48] One way to achieve this is through a better understanding of the alcohol risk-and-harm continuum.

Low-risk use

The U.S. National Institute of Alcohol Abuse and Alcoholism (NIAAA) initially recommended no more than two standard drinks (12 grams of pure alcohol per drink) per day for men and one standard drink per day for women.[49] More recently, they changed these recommendations in a physician's guide.[50] Men are at risk for alcohol-related problems if they drink more than 14 drinks in a week or more than four drinks on one occasion. Nonpregnant women are considered at risk if they drink more than seven drinks per week or more than three drinks on any one occasion.[50] Another guide for primary care clinicians also adopted these recommendations.[51]

The Alcohol Risk Assessment and Intervention Project, sponsored by the College of Family Physicians of Canada, also has developed guidelines for low-risk drinking.[52] According to their guidelines, men should not exceed four drinks and nonpregnant women should not exceed three drinks on any single day. No one should exceed 12 unit drinks (10 grams per drink) in a week.[53] In Britain, the Royal Colleges of General Practitioners, Psychiatrists, and Practitioners advised what they termed a "sensible" weekly limit of 21 small drinks (8 grams of pure alcohol per drink) for men and 14 for women.[54] More recently, a government publication from England raised the limits to 21 units for women and 28 units for men, despite objections from the medical profession.

As noted, marked variations exist internationally in terms of the amount of pure alcohol in a standard drink.[55] Furthermore, international differences exist with regard to alcohol use during pregnancy. In the United States, pregnant women are advised not to drink alcohol, whereas in England an occasional drink during pregnancy is not considered a significant risk.[56] Putting these controversial issues aside, the most important issue is for each country to define its own limit for low-risk drinking (see Table 4a.1 on the next page).

Table 4a.1 Low-risk Drinking Recommendations

Alcohol	Canada		U.S.		Britain/England	
	Men	Women	Men	Women	Men	Women
Standard drinks/week	12	12	14	7	28	21
Grams/drink	10	10	12	12	8	8
Total grams per week	120	120	168	84	224	168

Hazardous use

Hazardous use of alcohol is defined as drinking more than low-risk limits without evidence of harm or dependency. These patients are at increased risk for developing alcohol abuse and dependency, particularly if they increase their consumption over time.

Harmful use (abuse)

Harmful use of alcohol includes the diagnosis of alcohol abuse and is defined as drinking that causes any negative medical, psychological, and/or social consequences. A NIAAA alcohol alert publication compared the DSM-IV and ICD-10 classifications for alcohol abuse/harmful use (Table 4a.2).

Table 4a.2: DSM-IV and ICD-10 Definitions of Abuse (harmful use)
DSM-IV Alcohol Abuse
A. A maladaptive pattern of alcohol use leading to clinically significant impairment or distress, as manifested by one (or more) of the following occurring within a 12-month period: (1) recurrent drinking resulting in a failure to fulfill major role obligations at work, school, or home   (2) recurrent drinking in situations in which it is physically hazardous   (3) recurrent alcohol-related legal problems   (4) continued alcohol use despite having persistent or recurrent social or interpersonal problems caused or exacerbated by the effects of alcohol   B. The symptoms have never met the criteria for alcohol dependence.
ICD-10 Harmful Use of Alcohol
A. A pattern of alcohol use that is causing damage to health. The damage may be physical or mental. The diagnosis requires that actual damage should have been caused to the mental or physical health of the user.   B. No concurrent diagnosis of the alcohol dependence syndrome.

Dependency

The same NIAAA publication also compared DSM-IV and ICD-10 classifications for alcohol dependency (Table 4a.3). You also can use the 25-item Alcohol Dependence Scale instrument to assess the severity of alcohol dependence quantitatively.[57]

Table 4a.3: Definitions of Abuse and Dependence

	DSM-IV	ICD-10
Symptoms	A. A maladaptive pattern of alcohol use, leading to clinically significant impairment or distress, as manifested by three or more of the following occurring at any time in the same year:	A. Three or more of the following have been experienced or exhibited at some time during the previous year:
Tolerance	(1) Need for markedly increased amounts of alcohol to achieve intoxication or desired effect; or markedly diminished effect with continued use of the same amount of alcohol	(1) Evidence of tolerance, such that increased doses are required in order to achieve effects originally produced by lower doses
Withdrawal	(2) The characteristic withdrawal syndrome for alcohol; or alcohol (or a closely related substance) is taken to relieve or avoid withdrawal symptoms	(2) A physiological withdrawal state when drinking has ceased or been reduced, as evidenced by: the characteristic alcohol withdrawal syndrome, or use of alcohol (or a closely related substance) to relieve or avoid withdrawal symptoms
Impaired Control	(3) Persistent desire or one or more unsuccessful efforts to cut down or control drinking (4) Drinking in larger amounts or over a longer period than the person intended	(3) Difficulties in controlling drinking in terms of onset, termination, or levels of use
Neglect of Activities	(5) Important social, occupational, or recreational activities given up or reduced because of drinking	(4) Progressive neglect of alternative pleasures or interests in favor of drinking; or
Time Spent Drinking	(6) A great deal of time spent in activities necessary to obtain alcohol, to drink, or to recover from its effects	(5) A great deal of time spent in activities necessary to obtain alcohol, to drink, or to recover from its effects
Drinking Despite Problems	(7) Continued drinking despite knowledge of having a persistent or recurrent physical or physiological problem that is likely to be caused or exacerbated by alcohol use	(6) Continued drinking despite clear evidence of overtly harmful physical or psychological consequences
Compulsive Use	None	(7) A strong desire or sense of compulsion to drink
Duration Criterion	B. No duration criterion separately specified. However, three or more dependence criteria must be met within the same year and must occur repeatedly, as specified by duration qualifiers associated with criteria (e.g., "often," "persistent," "continued")	B. No duration criterion separately specified. However, three or more dependence criteria must be met during the previous year.
Criterion for Subtyping Dependence	With physiological dependence: Evidence of tolerance or withdrawal—i.e., any of items A(1) or A(2) above are present Without physiological dependence: No evidence of tolerance or withdrawal—i.e., none of items A(1) or A(2) above are present	None

B. Risk and Harm Reduction

Risk and harm reduction refers to lowering the severity of excessive alcohol use for individuals and populations at large with any of the following goals: reduced alcohol intake, low-risk drinking, or abstinence. This concept, which aims to reduce the overall percentage of patients who drink above low-risk limits, whatever their severity of excessive alcohol use, can be used to address many other risk behaviors. When it is not possible to achieve the ideal goal for change, you can use this concept to make an incremental reduction in risk and harm associated with any risk behavior.

C. The Challenge of Making a Definitive Diagnosis

In primary care and hospital settings, it is often difficult to conduct comprehensive assessments to make a definite diagnosis of alcohol abuse and/or dependence with confidence. One way is to make a diagnosis unilaterally, using a likelihood of at-risk and problem drinking scale ranging from unlikely to possible to probably to definitely (see Table 4a.4).[58] Such a scale can help you track how your and your patient's perceptions of risk differ. The following example is of a patient, Mr. A.

Making Tentative and Definitive Diagnoses — Mr. A. attended his routine physical exam, where MP (motivational practitioner) took an alcohol and drug history. Mr. A. stated that he smoked about 15 cigarettes a day and drank 20 beers on weekends. His only complaint was heartburn and indigestion on the weekend. Although Mr. A. did not view his drinking behavior as a problem, MP was concerned about the probability of alcohol abuse and possible alcohol dependency. To get a better understanding of how he and Mr. A. differed in their perceptions of risk and problem drinking, MP filled out Table 4a.4.

Commentary: Based on this partial assessment, MP established that the patient was definitely drinking above low-risk limits, even though Mr. A. did not view his drinking behavior as a health issue. This helped MP realize that his opinion differed from Mr. A's perspective.

Table 4a.4: Differences in Perspective about At-risk and Problem Drinking

Likelihood of a Problem	At-risk Drinker (Hazardous use)	Problem Drinker	
		Abuse	Dependency
Definitely	Pr		
Probably		Pr	
Possibly			Pr
Unlikely	Pt	Pt	Pt

Pr = Practitioner's opinion   Pt = Practitioner's opinion of Mr. A's perspective

Even if you are certain of a diagnosis, it is often challenging to inform patients in ways they will accept. Rather than taking full responsibility for making the diagnosis, you can share this responsibility with patients in ways that enable them to take an active role in the process.

Using uncertainty to make the diagnosis

Because of time constraints and diagnostic uncertainty, you may not always feel confident about diagnosing hazardous, harmful, and/or dependent use of alcohol. You can, however, educate patients by using a likelihood scale (possibly, probably, definitely) about their possible alcohol use (see Table 4a.5). This approach gives you the option of educating patients in a confident manner (using the word definitely) or in a tentative manner (using the word possibly) for a variety of diagnoses. This approach is an alternative strategy to making the diagnosis unilaterally *and* telling patients about it.

Table 4a.5: Using the Likelihood Scale to Educate Patients about their Alcohol Use*
For hazardous drinking – *"I'm concerned that you are (possibly, probably, definitely) drinking above what are considered to be low-risk limits. What do you think?"* [Let the patient respond.]
For harmful drinking – *"I'm concerned that your health (possibly, probably, definitely) may be caused or made worse by alcohol. What do you think?"* [Let the patient respond.]
For alcohol dependence – *"I'm concerned that you are (possibly, probably, definitely) dependent upon alcohol (or have built up a tolerance to the effects of alcohol because . . .). What do you think?"* [Let the patient respond.]

*Reproduced with permission.[58]

Using the likelihood scale, you can educate patients about the severity of at-risk (hazardous use) or problem drinking in a nonthreatening way. For example, "The amount that you are drinking is definitely above low-risk limits. What I'm concerned about is that your alcohol is probably causing your high blood pressure, and you could possibly be dependent on alcohol without knowing it." It is often easier to reach a consensus with patients about at-risk drinking than it is to gain agreement about alcohol abuse and dependence. Some patients are truly surprised that they drink more than most of the population. They may doubt, resist, and resent even a tentative diagnosis of alcohol abuse or dependence. Rather than arguing about the diagnosis, you can educate and help patients better understand how their drinking habit is affecting their health. Alternatively, you can show patients and their families the diagnostic criteria of abuse and dependency and let them deal with the discrepancy between their opinion and professional opinion.

Dealing with Diagnostic Uncertainty—After doing a partial assessment, MP thought that Mr. A. definitely drank above low-risk limits, probably was abusing alcohol, and possibly was dependent on alcohol; he also felt that Mr. A. would deny any of these diagnostic possibilities. MP first educated Mr. A. about low-risk drinking limits, shared his definitive diagnosis (hazardous use of alcohol) with Mr. A., and then asked Mr. A. what he thought about it. Mr. A. was surprised by this information because many of his friends drank even more than he did. MP explained that both Mr. A.'s and his friends' drinking habits were well above average. Mr. A.

listened to his practitioner's reasons for raising the issue of low-risk drinking and agreed that he probably drank too much, given the definition of low-risk drinking (i.e., 14 standard drinks per week and no more than four drinks on any one occasion). Mr. A. was also willing to accept that alcohol was possibly making his indigestion and heartburn worse. Since MP did not yet have sufficient information to justify his concerns about the possibility of alcohol dependency, he did not raise this issue at this appointment. However, MP did establish more of a common understanding with Mr. A. about hazardous and harmful use of alcohol.

Commentary: By using the likelihood scale to discuss Mr. A.'s excessive drinking, MP was able to track how Mr. A. shifted in his understanding about the severity of at-risk and problem drinking (see Table 4a.6). You can use this table as well to track the extent to which you and your patients share similar perceptions about the likelihood for at-risk and problem drinking.

Table 4a.6: Enhancing Mutual Understanding about At-risk and Problem Drinking

Likelihood of a Problem	At-risk Drinker (Hazardous use)	Problem Drinker	
		Abuse	Dependency
Definitely			
Probably	C		
Possibly		C	*Pr*
Unlikely			*Pt*

C = Common agreement between practitioner and patient
Pr = Practitioner's opinion
Pt = Patient's opinion

If you work too quickly, however, or are too forceful, some patients will resist accepting your educational message. To avoid such resistance, you can use an indirect approach that involves patients in a process of negotiating a common understanding about the diagnosis before moving on to the issue of alcohol dependency. For example, "Your drinking is above low-risk limits, and there is a possibility that it could be causing your high blood pressure." You can then invite the patient to do a trial of abstinence to see if blood pressure goes down and assess for any withdrawal symptoms before addressing the topic of alcohol dependence. As is described in Chapter 4b, you can even show patients the criteria for the diagnosis and invite them to give their opinion about how these criteria relate to them.

MOVING ON

You can use diagnostic uncertainty and the alcohol risk-and-harm continuum to negotiate with patients about excessive alcohol use. These skills, steps 3 and 4 (assessment and enhancing mutual understanding) of the six-step approach, are described in the next chapter, which explains how you can work with patients over time to reduce their alcohol risk and harms.

Web sites for Practitioners and Patients

National Institute on Alcohol Abuse and Alcoholism has a wealth of resources available on line http://www.niaaa.nih.gov/, including Alcohol alerts, http://www.niaaa.nih.gov/publications/aa43.htm.

The National Institute of Drug Abuse http://www.nida.nih.gov/ is a resource of information for researchers, health care professionals, teachers and students.

SAMHSA's National Clearinghouse for Alcohol and Drug Information http://www.health.org/ has drug and information facts sheets and hyperlinks to a variety of drug information Web sites.

NCADI Research Briefs on Alcohol and Substance Abuse: http://www.health.org/res-brf/Rbriefs.htm

National Center on Addiction and Substance Abuse http://www.casacolumbia.org/ is a unique think/action tank that engages all disciplines to study every form of substance abuse as it affects our society.

Alcohol and Drug Institute (Washington, U.S.A.) http://depts.washington.edu/adai/ supports and facilitates research and research dissemination in the field of alcohol and drug abuse.

Center for Alcoholism, Substance Abuse and Addiction http://casaa-0031.unm.edu/links.html disseminates new knowledge on alcoholism, substance abuse, and other addictive behaviors and fosters communication and collaboration among researchers in multiple disciplines, and between researchers and those in applied areas. Enhances motivation for change in substance abuse treatment. Miller, W. R. (Ed.) (1999). Treatment Improvement Protocol (TIP) Series, No. 35. Rockville, MD: Center for Substance Abuse Treatment. Download from this site: http://text.nlm.nih.gov/ftrs/pick?ftrsK=46325&cd=1&t=951249244&collect=tip&dbName=tip35

Alcohol Concern www.alcoholconcern.org.uk has extensive listing of many other alcohol-related Web sites. Go to http://www.alcoholconcern.org.uk/Links/Alcohol_Links.htm

Alcohol Education and Research Council www.aerc.org.uk seeks to increase awareness of alcohol issues and to facilitate a reduction in alcohol-related harm in society.

Medical Council on Alcoholism: www.medicouncilalcol.demon.co.uk is committed to improving medical understanding of alcohol-related problems.

Community Drug Education Project http://www.drugsinfo.org.uk/www_links.htm has a list of related Web sites.

World Health Organization Collaborative Project on Identification and Management of Alcohol-related Problems in Primary Health Care (Phase IV) has a description of its activities at http://www.alcohol-phaseivproject.co.uk/

Addiction search http://www.addictionsearch.com/ provides gateway to research-based addiction information for health consumers, health professionals, educators, students, and researchers.

Web of Addictions http://www.well.com/user/woa/index.html is dedicated to providing accurate information about alcohol and other drug addictions.

Centre for Addiction & Mental Health (Canada) http://www.camh.net/ has been designated a WHO Center for Excellence. Provides a wealth of resources for professional and lay audiences.

Canadian Centre on Substance Abuse http://www.ccsa.ca/ is a non-profit organization working to minimize the harm associated with the use of alcohol, tobacco and other drugs.

Health Care Information Resources http://www-hsl.mcmaster.ca/tomflem/addict.html makes information about health and disease accessible in the belief that the informed consumer is a more satisfied consumer of health care.

National Drug and Alcohol Center (Australia) http://www.med.unsw.edu.au/ndarc/ increases the effectiveness of combatting alcohol and drug problems in Australia.

National Drug Research Institute (Australia) http://www.curtin.edu.au/curtin/centre/ndri/ works to prevent harmful drug use in Australia.

Substance abuse http://www.yourhealthlinks.com/substanceabuse/substanceabuse.html has a comprehensive list of additional Web sites.

Cyber-Psych http://www.cyber-psych.com/addict.html has a site for the general public about addictions

About.com Alcoholism http://alcoholism.about.com/health/alcoholism/mbody.htm?COB=home provides a guide to over 700 Web sites and news items about alcoholism.

Guided Self-change clinic http://www.nova.edu/~gsc/ helps problem drinkers change.

Recreational Drugs Information Homepage http://www.a1b2c3.com/drugs/index.htm lists and describes a wide variety of drugs used.

Center for On-Line Addiction http://www.netaddiction.com/ provides help and resources on the Internet to addicts, health care professionals and corporations.

Recovery Liberation Front http://www.aahorror.net/Home.htm addresses the issues of harm caused by the misuse of the 12-step AA approach.

Reference List

1. Pirmohamed M, Gilmore IT. Alcohol abuse and the burden on the NHS—time for action. J R Coll Physicians 2000;34: 161-162

2. Secretary of Health and Human Services. Eighth Special Report to the U.S. Congress on Alcohol and Health. 1993. Arlington, Va., Dept. of Health and Human Services.

3. Buchsbaum DG, Buchanan RG, Lawton MJ, et al. Alcohol consumption patterns in a primary care population. Alcohol and Alcoholism 1991;26: 215-220

4. Magruder-Habib K, Durand AM, Frey KA. Alcohol abuse and alcoholism in primary health care settings. J Fam Pract 1991;32: 406-413

5. Leckman AL, Umland BE, Blay M. Prevalence of alcoholism in a family practice center. J Fam Pract 1984;18: 867-870

6. Hill A, Rumpf HJ, Hapke U, et al. Prevalence of alcohol dependence and abuse in general practice. Alcohol Clin Exp Res 1998;22: 935-940

7. Burge SK, Schneider FD. Alcohol-related problems: recognition and intervention. Am Fam Physician 1999;59: 361-70, 372

8. Buchsbaum DG, Buchanan RG, Poses RM, et al. Physician detection of drinking problems in patients attending a general medicine practice. J Gen Intern Med 1992;7: 517-521

9. Cleary PD, Miller M, Bush BT, et al. Prevalence and recognition of alcohol abuse in a primary care population. American Journal of Medicine 1988;85: 466-471

10. Nuffield Institute for Health, University of Leeds, Centre for Health Economics, University of York, Research Unit, and Royal College of Physicians. Effective health care: Brief interventions and alcohol use. 7. 1993. The Department of Health.

11. Bien TH, Miller WR, Tonigan JS. Brief interventions for alcohol problems: A review. Addiction 1993;88(3): 315-335

12. Kahan M, Wilson L, Becker L. Effectiveness of physician-based interventions with problem drinkers: A review. Canadian Medical Association Journal 1995;152(6): 851-859

13. McAvoy BR. Alcohol education for general practitioners in the United Kingdom. Alcohol and Alcoholism 2000;35: 225-229

14. Wallace P. Patients with alcohol problems—simple questioning is the key to effective identification and management (Editorial). British Journal of General Practice 2001;51: 172-173

15. Lawlor DA, Keen S, Neal RD. Can general practitioners influence the nation's health through a population approach to provision of lifestyle advice? Br J Gen Pract 2000;50: 455-459

16. Deehan A, Marshall EJ, Strang J. Tackling alcohol misuse: opportunities and obstacles in primary care. Br J Gen Pract 1998;48: 1779-1782

17. Kristenson H, Ohlin H, Hultën-Nosslin MB, et al. Identification and intervention of heavy drinking in middle-aged men: Results and follow-up of 24-60 months of long-term study with randomized controls. Alcoholism: Clinical and Experimental Research 1983;7: 203-209

18. Anderson P. Effectiveness of general practice interventions for patients with harmful alcohol consumption. Br J Gen Pract 1993;43: 386-389

19. Anderson P, Scott E. The effect of general practitioners' advice to heavy drinking men. Br J Addict 1992;87: 891-900

20. Walsh DC, Hingson RW, Merrigan DM, et al. A randomized trial of treatment options for alcohol-abusing workers. New England Journal of Medicine 1991;325: 775-782

21. Persson J, Magnusson PH. Prevalence of excessive or problem drinkers among patients attending somatic outpatient clinics: A study of alcohol related medical care. British Medical Journal—Clinical Research 1987;295: 467-472

22. Persson J, Magnusson PH. Sickness, absenteeism and mortality in patients with excessive drinking in somatic out-patient care. Scandinavian Journal of Primary Health Care 1989;7: 211-217

23. Wallace P, Cutler S, Haines A. Randomized controlled trial of general practitioner intervention in patients with excessive alcohol consumption. British Medical Journal 1988;297: 663-668

24. Babor TF, Grant M. WHO Collaborating Investigators Project on identification and management of alcohol-related problems. Combined analyses of outcome data: The cross-national generalizability of brief interventions. Report on phase II: A randomized clinical trial of brief interventions in primary health care. Copenhagen: WHO; 1992

25. Magruder-Habib K, Durand AM, Frey KA. Alcohol abuse and alcoholism in primary health care settings. The Journal of Family Practice 1991;32: 406-413

26. Heather N, Rollnick S, Bell A, et al. Effects of brief counselling among male heavy drinkers identified on general hospital wards. Drug and Alcohol Review 1996;15: 29-38

27. Anderson P, Scott E. The effect of general practitioners' advice to heavy drinking men. British Journal of Addiction 1992;87: 891-900

28. Romelsjo A, Andersson L, Barrner H, et al. A randomized study of secondary prevention of early stage problem drinkers in primary health care. Br J Addict 1989;84: 1319-1327

29. Cowan PF. An intervention to improve the assessment of alcoholism by practicing physicians. Fam Pract Res J 1994;14: 41-49

30. Chick J, Lloyd G, Crombie E. Counselling problem drinkers in medical wards: A controlled study. British Medical Journal—Clinical Research 1985;290: 965-967

31. Maheswaran R, Beevers M, Beevers DG. Effectiveness of advice to reduce alcohol consumption in hypertensive patients. Hypertension 1992;19(1): 79-84

32. WHO Brief Intervention Study Group. A cross-national trial of brief interventions with heavy drinkers. American Journal of Public Health 1996;86: 948-955

33. Fleming MF, Barry KL, Manwell LB, et al. Brief physician advice for problem alcohol drinkers: A randomized controlled trial in community-based primary care practices. JAMA 1997;277: 1039-1045

34. Wallace P, Cremona A, Anderson P. Safe limits of drinking: General practitioners' views. British Medical Journal—Clinical Research 1985;290(6485): 1875-1876

35. Klatsky AL. Annotation: Alcohol and longevity. American Journal of Public Health 1995;85: 16-18

36. Pearson TA, Terry P. What to advise patients about drinking alcohol. JAMA 1994;272: 957-958

37. Donahue RP, Abbott RD. Alcohol and haemorrhagic stroke [letter]. Lancet 1986;2: 515-516

38. Stampfer MJ, Colditz GA, Willett WC, et al. A prospective study of moderate alcohol consumption and the risk of coronary disease and stroke in women. New England Journal of Medicine 1988;319: 267-273

39. Klatsky AL, Armstrong MA, Friedman GD. Alcohol and stroke. Journal of the American College of Cardiology 1987;9: 78A

40. Tanaka H, Ueda Y, Hayashi M, et al. Risk factors for cerebral hemorrhage and cerebral infarction in a Japanese rural community. Stroke 1982;13: 62-73

41. Institute of Medicine. Broadening the base of treatment for alcohol problems. Washington, D.C.: National Academy Press; 1990

42. Skinner HA. Spectrum of drinkers and intervention opportunities. Canadian Medical Association Journal 1990;143: 1054-1059

43. Cahalan D. Problem drinkers: A national survey. San Francisco: Jossey-Bass; 1970

44. Archer L, Grant BF, Dawson DA. What if Americans drank less? The potential effect on the prevalence of alcohol abuse and dependence. American Journal of Public Health 1995;85: 61-66

45. Kreitman N. Alcohol consumption and the preventive paradox. British Journal of Addiction 1986;81: 353-363

46. Rose G. Sick individuals and sick populations. International Journal of Epidemiology 1985;14(1): 32-38

47. Kendell RE. The physician's role. Canadian Medical Association Journal 1990;143: 1042-1047

48. Anderson P. Management of alcohol problems: The role of the general practitioner. Alcohol & Alcoholism 1993;28(3): 263-272

49. U.S. Department of Health & Human Services. Moderate drinking. Alcohol Alert: National Institute on Alcohol Abuse and Alcoholism 1992;16(PH315): 1-4

50. National Institute on Alcohol Abuse and Alcoholism. Fourth Special Report to the U.S. Congress on Alcohol and Health. U.S. Department of Health and Human Services. 1981.

51. Center for Substance Abuse Treatment. A guide to substance abuse services for primary care clinicians. No. 24. Treatment Improvement Protocol (TIP) Series. 1997. Substance Abuse and Mental Health Services Administration.

52. Peters C, Wilson D, Bruneau A, et al. Alcohol risk assessment and intervention for family physicians. Canadian Family Physician 1996;42: 681-689

53. Sanchez-Craig M, Wilkinson DA, Davila R. How much is too much? Further evaluation of empirically-based guidelines for moderate drinking: One-year results of three studies with male and female problem drinkers. Toronto: Addiction Research Foundation; 1994

54. Lord President's report on action against alcohol misuse. London, England: Her Majesty's Stationery Office; 1991

55. Miller WR, Heather N, Hall W. Calculating standard drink units: International comparisons. British Journal of Addiction 1991;86(1): 43-47

56. Knupfer G. Abstaining for foetal health: The fiction that even light drinking is dangerous. British Journal of Addiction 1991;86: 1063-1073

57. Ross HE, Gavin DR, Skinner HA. Diagnostic validity of the MAST and the alcohol dependence scale in the assessment of DSM-III alcohol disorders. Journal of Studies on Alcohol 1990;51: 506-513

58. Botelho RJ, Novak S. Dealing with Substance Misuse, Abuse and Dependency. Primary Care 1993;20: 51-70

CHAPTER 4b

REDUCING ALCOHOL RISK AND HARM

FOR REFLECTION

How do you deal with patients who do not respond to your advice to keep below the low-risk drinking limit or to abstain from alcohol use?

OVERVIEW

About 20% of patients who drink excessive amounts of alcohol will respond to health education and advice to reduce alcohol consumption to below low-risk limits. Even when patients have alcohol-related complications, however, they will not respond to your advice to change. Furthermore, many patients are dependent on alcohol without your knowing about it. This chapter will help you learn how to deal with the full spectrum of resistant patients who have a hazardous, harmful, and dependent use of alcohol; it can also help you work with patients who drink and drive, request sedative drugs, and/or provide rationalizations to avoid dealing with their excessive alcohol use.

REDUCING ALCOHOL RISK AND HARM

To learn new skills, first work with patients who drink above low-risk limits or have alcohol-related problems. After you have developed some skills, you can learn how to deal with patients with alcohol dependence.

STEP 1: BUILDING PARTNERSHIPS

You can build your partnership with patients throughout the problem-solving process. For example, you can use the decision balance in ways that strengthen your partnership with patients and thereby enhance the prospects of facilitating change.

A. Develop Empathy
You can use a variety of communication skills to develop empathy with patients. Practitioners who develop higher levels of empathy with patients, even at the first encounter, are more successful in helping patients reduce their alcohol intake. [1-4]

Communication Skills for Developing Empathy	
Use open-ended questions	*"So, what is your favorite drink?"*
Use reflective listening	*"So, alcohol helps you relax and deal with your fears."*
Paraphrase	*"You have difficulty understanding where those fears come from."*
Validate feelings	*"These fears are overwhelming and make life difficult for you."*
Normalize behaviors	*"It's normal to have fears and want them to go away."*
Affirm strengths	*"It takes courage to understand and come to terms with those fears."*
Use probing questions	*"When do those fears occur? What do you fear from your past? What fears do you have now and for the future?"*

B. Use Relational Skills Effectively
At any problem-solving step, you can take the one-down position with the patient or put the patient in a one-up position. For example, you can use these relational skills during step 4 (enhancing mutual understanding) when patients resist the notion that they drink excessively.

Putting the Patient in the One-up Position
"Tell me what convinces you that you do not have an alcohol-related problem." *"How would you know whether you are dependent on alcohol?"* *"Tell me what would convince you that you have an alcohol-related problem."* *"Is there anything that would convince you that you are dependent on alcohol?"* *"What would have to happen to convince you that you need to change?"*
Taking the One-down Position with a Patient
"I'm not sure what it would take for you to think that you may have an alcohol-related problem or are dependent on alcohol." *"I'm not sure what you would like to know about alcohol-related problems or alcohol dependency that would be helpful to you."* *"I'm not sure what it would take to convince you about the need to keep to low-risk drinking, or abstain from alcohol."*

C. Clarify Roles and Responsibilities

More often than not, you and your patients assume roles and responsibilities without any explicit negotiation. The option of explicitly clarifying your roles and responsibilities with your patients is appropriate before the agenda-setting step, but you can use this option at any time, particularly when patient resistance occurs.

Clarifying Your Roles
Clarify your prevention role: *"Alcohol can damage your health before you get any symptoms. You can prevent problems before they occur. Can we do a checkup to see if alcohol is damaging your health in any way?"* Motivational role (treating alcohol abuse): *"I can always treat your bouts of pancreatitis (or any other alcohol-related problem), but you seem undecided about whether to stop drinking. Would you like me to help you develop the motivation to quit drinking?"*
Clarifying Responsibility
"I'll tell you what I know about the risks and harmful effects related to your alcohol use. I suspect we see the benefits, risks, and harm of alcohol use in different ways. As long as we see them differently, we may have some difficulties in trying to improve your health. Perhaps we can put our differences to work for us rather than against us."

STEP 2: NEGOTIATING AN AGENDA

You can either use a prevention-focused or problem-focused approach to negotiate an agenda with patients about assessing their pattern of alcohol use. After gathering sufficient information to suspect hazardous, harmful, or dependent use of alcohol, you can proceed to conduct an assessment.

A. Prevention-focused Approach

The following options can help you identify at-risk patients or hazardous drinkers who do not have any alcohol-related problems.

Use direct questions about alcohol and drug use

Direct questions (closed-ended or open-ended) represent the traditional way of obtaining a history of substance abuse; for example, "How many drinks do you have in a week?" When asked direct questions, some patients show signs of resistance. This cue may increase your suspicion of an underlying drinking problem. Sometimes, attempts to quantify alcohol consumption make patients less likely to cooperate. In such circumstances, you may choose not to pursue an accurate alcohol history, but instead opt for leading or screening questions and/or conducting an assessment.

Consent-gaining Direct Questions
About health: *"I'd like to check whether there is anything you can do to improve your health. Is that all right?"* [Let patient respond.] You can then ask, *"Do you drink alcohol?" "What kinds of alcohol do you drink? Beer, wine, hard liquor?" "Do you drink daily? How many drinks do you have in a week?" "What size drinks do you usually have?" "How much beer, wine, or hard liquor do you buy in a week?"*

Use leading questions

As some drinkers are vague in quantifying their alcohol use, leading questions may help you obtain a more accurate history. These questions assume that people enjoy drinking alcohol.

Using Leading Questions to Detect Excessive Alcohol Use—Mr. A., age 85, was admitted to the emergency room with chest pains. He admitted to the emergency room physician that he smoked three packs of cigarettes a day and drank one beer a day. He was diagnosed as having unstable angina with electrocardiogram changes suggestive of an evolving myocardial infarction. After Mr. A. was given thrombolytic therapy, his attending physician visited him in the emergency room to assess his risk for alcohol withdrawal syndrome because his family stated that he drank a lot. He asked Mr. A., "What is your favorite beer?" Mr. A. smiled and mentioned the brand name of an inexpensive beer. The attending physician continued, "How many beers a day do you like to drink?" "Oh, maybe five or six beers a day," replied the patient.

Leading Open-ended Questions
"So, what kinds of alcohol do you like to drink?" "What are your favorite drinks?" "What do you like to drink when you go out to a party?"

Administer screening questionnaires

The CAGE questionnaire (see Table 4b.1 on the next page) is the briefest instrument for detecting past and present alcohol abuse and/or dependence, but is not appropriate for detecting hazardous use of alcohol.[5;6] If you have not used the CAGE questionnaire before, you may feel awkward using it with patients. Prefacing statements can help to reduce your feeling of awkwardness and prepare patients for these questions: for example, "I would like to ask you a few questions about how alcohol is affecting your health. Is that okay?" Alternatively, you may intersperse these questions during your conversations with patients, rather than asking them in a sequential manner.

The sensitivity of the CAGE questionnaire ranges from 49%-89% and specificity from 79%-95%.[7-11] Therefore, a negative response on this questionnaire will still miss many patients who have a problem of harmful use of alcohol, as well as the majority of patients who have a hazardous use of alcohol. Patients with a negative screen on the CAGE questionnaire may still require an assessment if they present with complaints that may be associated with alcohol use, or if they drink more than the low-risk drinking limit.

Table 4b.1: CAGE Questionnaire	
C	*"Have you ever felt you should Cut down on your drinking?"*
A	*"Has anyone Annoyed you by criticizing your drinking?"*
G	*"Have you ever felt bad or Guilty about your drinking?"*
E	*"Have you ever had a drink (an Eye opener) first thing in the morning to steady your nerves or to get rid of a hangover?"*
Decision rule: Two or more positive responses may indicate alcohol abuse or dependence. One positive response warrants further assessment.	

Another screening instrument is the 10-item Audit questionnaire (see Table 4b.2 on the next page) developed by the World Health Organization Early Intervention Project for use in primary care.[12-16] This instrument has an advantage over the CAGE questionnaire in that you can identify both hazardous and problem drinkers (alcohol abuse and dependence).

Table 4b.2: Audit Questionnaire

Please check the answer to each question that is correct for you:

1. How often do you have a drink containing alcohol?
❑ Never ❑ Monthly or less ❑ Two to four times a month ❑ Two to three times a week ❑ Four or more times a week

2. How many drinks containing alcohol do you have on a typical day when you are drinking?
❑ 1 or 2 ❑ 3 or 4 ❑ 5 or 6 ❑ 7 to 9 ❑ 10 or more

3. How often do you have six or more drinks on one occasion?
❑ Never ❑ Less than monthly ❑ Monthly ❑ Weekly ❑ Daily or almost daily

4. How often during the last year have you found that you were not able to stop drinking once you had started?
❑ Never ❑ Less than monthly ❑ Monthly ❑ Weekly ❑ Daily or almost daily

5. How often during the last year have you failed to do what was normally expected from you because of drinking?
❑ Never ❑ Less than monthly ❑ Monthly ❑ Weekly ❑ Daily or almost daily

6. How often during the last year have you needed a first drink in the morning to get yourself going after a heavy drinking session?
❑ Never ❑ Less than monthly ❑ Monthly ❑ Weekly ❑ Daily or almost daily

7. How often during the last year have you had a feeling of guilt or remorse after drinking?
❑ Never ❑ Less than monthly ❑ Monthly ❑ Weekly ❑ Daily or almost daily

8. How often during the last year have you been unable to remember what happened the night before because you had been drinking?
❑ Never ❑ Less than monthly ❑ Monthly ❑ Weekly ❑ Daily or almost daily

9. Have you or someone else been injured as a result of your drinking?
❑ No ❑ Yes, but not in the last year ❑ Yes, during the last year

10. Has a relative, friend, doctor, or other health worker been concerned about your drinking or suggested you cut down?
❑ No ❑ Yes, but not in the last year ❑ Yes, during the last year

Questions 1-8 are scored 0-4 points, and questions 9-10 are scored 0, 2 or 4 points, giving a possible range of 0-40 points.

Patients can complete the AUDIT instrument themselves; given its length, it is unlikely to be used commonly during routine patient encounters. The AUDIT-C (consumption) instrument has been developed. This shortened version consists of the first three questions listed above, giving a possible range score of 0-12.[15] Another instrument, the Five-shot Questionnaire (see Table 4b.3 on the next page), has been developed to meet the need for brevity.[17]

Table 4b.3: Five-shot Questionnaire

Please check the answer to each question that is correct for you:				
1. How often do you have a drink containing alcohol?				
❏ Never	❏ Monthly or less	❏ Two to four times a month	❏ Two to three times a week	❏ Four or more times a week
2. How many drinks containing alcohol do you have on a typical day when you are drinking?				
❏ 1 or 2	❏ 3 or 4	❏ 5 or 6	❏ 7 to 9	❏ 10 or more
3. Have people annoyed you by criticizing your drinking?			❏ No	❏ Yes
4. Have you ever felt bad or guilty about your drinking?			❏ No	❏ Yes
5. Have you ever had a drink first thing in the morning to steady your nerves or to get rid of a hangover?			❏ No	❏ Yes

Questions 1 and 2 are scored 0-0.5-1.0-1.5-2.0 points, and questions 3-5 are scored 0-1, giving a possible range of 0-7 points.

A study compared the screening properties of these instruments for detecting alcohol abuse or dependence in general practice (see Table 4b.4).[18] The Audit-C and Five-shot questionnaires both performed well in terms of sensitivity and specificity for men. In women, the Five-shot Questionnaire has superior sensitivity rates over the Audit-C, but the reverse was true for specificity.

Table 4b.4: Performance of Screening Tests in General Practice

Screening Test		Males		Females	
		Sensitivity	Specificity	Sensitivity	Specificity
Cage	2 or >	47.7	92.3	37	96.8
Audit	5 or >	82.6	72.9	65.2	91.9
	6 or >	74.2	81.4	58.7	95.9
	8 or >	60.6	90.3	50.0	98.7
Audit-C	5 or >	78.0	74.9	50.0	93.2
	6 or >	66.7	84.3	39.1	97.3
	8 or >	48.5	94.3	21.7	99.6
Five-shot	2 or >	86.4	63.6	67.4	87.4
	2.5 or >	74.2	80.9	63.0	94.7
	3.0 or >	62.1	88.3	37.0	97.3

Other attempts have also been made to identify one or two screening questions instead of using questionnaires.[19-21] Based on the National Health Interview Survey, self-report of five or more drinks on one occasion over the past year had a sensitivity/specificity of 0.90/0.53 in men and 0.77/0.77 in women for alcohol abuse and dependence.[22;23] This question (modified to five or more drinks in the last three months) had a sensitivity of 62% and a specificity of 93% in primary care.[21] A positive result tripled the probability of problem drinking from 25% prevalence to a post-test probability of 74%, while a negative test reduced this probability from 25% to 12%.

Take a family history

The purpose of taking a family history for alcohol and drug problems is to identify and help high-risk patients as well as family members. Patients who come from families with a history of substance abuse are at increased risk of developing alcohol and drug problems. Family, twin, half-sibling, and adoption studies of alcoholic subjects suggest that the risk of inheritance of alcoholism is at least 50%.[24] The questions below can identify other family members who have drug or alcohol problems. For those patients whose family members have current alcohol or drug problems, you can encourage their relatives to seek professional help as well.

Screening for Alcohol and Drug Problems in the Family
"Has anyone in your family had alcohol or drug problems in the past?" *"Do you think anyone in your family has an alcohol or drug problem now?"* *"Can they drink more alcohol than most people and not get drunk?"*

B. Problem-focused Approach

Even if the outcome of the CAGE screening is negative, the following complaints are cues to possible alcohol related-problems:

- Medical: Injuries, gastrointestinal symptoms (dyspepsia, peptic ulcer, diarrhea), high blood pressure, minor and major accidents, chronic fatigue, headaches, back pain/chronic pain
- Psychological: Sleep problems, anxiety, depression, relationship difficulties, sexual problems
- Social: Poor work performance, poor school performance, missing work, loss of jobs, family problems, financial problems
- Legal: Driving while impaired or intoxicated; debts

Prefacing statements and exploratory questions help you to explore how patients view the association between their presenting problems and alcohol use.

Prefacing statements

Prefacing statements link the use of alcohol to patients' presenting complaints in ways that provide a rationale for taking an alcohol history, administering the CAGE questionnaire, or conducting an assessment.

Prefacing Statements
Normalizing and validating comments: *"Many people find that drinking alcohol helps them get to sleep. Is that how it is for you? Let me explain how alcohol causes poor sleep even though it helps you to get off to sleep."*
Comments that focus on concerns about the consequences: *"Some people find that drinking alcohol makes their stomach pain worse. Has that happened to you?" "Did you know that alcohol can cause high blood pressure?"*

Use exploratory questions

Exploratory questions help you engage patients in assessing how their health problems relate to their alcohol use. They include closed-ended linear questions, open-ended linear questions, and circular questions, as well as rephrasing prefacing statements as questions.

Exploratory Questions
Closed-ended linear questions: *"Has drinking alcohol made your stomach problem worse or better? Has your stomach problem affected how much you drink?" "Has drinking alcohol made your depression worse?"*
Open-ended linear questions: *"How has your drinking affected your health? How have concerns about your health affected how much you drink?" "In what ways has your drinking affected your depression?"*
Rephrase prefacing statements as questions: *"How does drinking alcohol affect your sleep?" "How does alcohol affect your depression?" "How is your sleeping problem affected by your use of alcohol?" "How does drinking help to reduce your blood pressure level?"*
Circular question: *"What concerns your family (spouse or children) about how your drinking affects your health?"*

STEP 3: ASSESSING RESISTANCE AND MOTIVATION

Depending on your patient's responses to negotiating an agenda, you can choose from an array of options to conduct motivational and disease-centered assessments. The distinctions between these assessments highlight some of the ways in which specialists and generalists deal with alcohol-related problems (see Table 4b.5). Patients who have a high probability of severe alcohol problems are often referred to specialists, who then conduct lengthy assessments and work with patients intensively for a limited period of time. Specialists diagnose a variety of medical, psychological, and social problems, and develop an appropriate management plan.

In contrast, generalists encounter patients who may be anywhere along the risk-and-harm continuum. They are often uncertain about the underlying severity of a patient's alcohol problem. A definitive diagnosis may take time.

Table 4b.5: Comparing Specialist and Generalist Assessments

Addiction Specialists	Practitioners
Referred patients	Case-finding
Standardized questionnaires and structured interviews	Individualized interviews using brief assessments
Organized, intensive program provided episodically in times of greatest need	Continuity of care provided in context of comprehensive, coordinated care
Linear, medical, or psychiatric assessments	Circular, behavioral assessments
Time-limited (hours)	Brief and recurrent (minutes)
Make a diagnosis & educate patients about it	Negotiate about a diagnosis

A. Motivational Assessment

To conduct a motivational assessment, you may use any of the following options: decision balance, readiness to initiate change, motivational reasons for change, energy to change, self-efficacy, and supports and barriers. As part of this process, you may also uncover psychiatric and psychological problems (anxiety disorders, depression, emotional disorders, suicidal ideation and intentions, and relationship problems), social problems (financial and work issues), legal problems (drinking while intoxicated) and medical problems (indigestion caused by alcohol).

Ask about readiness to change

Before using a decision balance, ask about the patient's readiness to change. The patient's response will help you decide whether to provide a stage-specific rationale. Furthermore, you can repeat questions about readiness to change to monitor a patient's progress over time.

Readiness to Change—Direct Questions
"Where are you in terms of dealing with cutting down to low-risk drinking (or quitting)?" [You can select one of the following three questions, or sequence them according to your impression of the patient.] *"Are you not interested in changing your drinking habit?"* *"Are you thinking about low-risk drinking or quitting?"* *"Are you willing to keep to low-risk drinking or stop drinking?"*
Readiness to Change—Indirect Questions
Consider any of the following: *"What do you think might convince you to keep to low-risk drinking?"* *"Do you think that you will ever cut down or quit drinking?"* *"When might you give up smoking?"* *"What, if anything, would help you decide to stop your binge drinking?"*

Use a decision balance with the patient

A stage-specific rationale helps patients understand why you are using the decision balance, particularly for those patients in precontemplation and in contemplation; first provide an appropriate rationale, and then show the patient what a decision balance looks like.

Providing Stage-specific Rationale and Gain Consent to Use the Decision Balance
Precontemplation: *"You told me about your stomach problem (or any other alcohol-related problem), and it may be made worse by drinking alcohol. Would you mind if we did a decision balance together to help you think about whether to change the amount of alcohol you drink?"*
Contemplation: *"You told me that you are thinking about changing the amount of alcohol that you drink. Would you mind if we did a decision balance together to help you decide whether to cut down to low-risk drinking limits (or abstain)?"*
Preparation: *"You think you will change soon. If we did a decision balance together, it could help you set a date to change. Is that okay?"*
Action: *"You are ready to set a date to change. If we did a decision balance together, it could help you prevent a relapse once you cut down or stop drinking."*

Showing the Decision Balance to the Patient
"Let me show you what a decision balance looks like. As we use the decision balance, it can help you understand better your reasons to stay the same and your reasons to consider change. But first [pointing to the right column], what you do you like about drinking alcohol? I would like to make a note of what you say. Is that okay? You can keep this decision balance to use when you go home, if you like."

After gaining the patient's cooperation in doing this task, you can ask one or more questions from each quadrant, preferably in the sequence suggested in the table below, or alter it to adapt to the patient's needs.

	Decision Balance	
Risk behavior	*1. Benefits* "What do you like about drinking alcohol?"	*2. Concerns* "Do you have any concerns about how alcohol affects your life?" "What concerns do you have about how alcohol affects your family or work?"
Reducing risk and harm	*3. Concerns* "What concerns would you have if you were to keep to low-risk drinking limits (or abstain)?" "In what way would your life be different if you were to quit for two weeks or longer?"	*4. Benefits* "In what ways would your health be better if you were to stop drinking or cut down?" "In what ways would other aspects of your life be better if you were to stop drinking or cut down?"

After completing the decision balance (see next page), give a copy with the responses to the patient and keep a copy of it in the patient's records. Alternatively, you can ask patients to complete this task in the waiting room or as a homework assignment for the next visit, perhaps with the input of a family member. At follow-up appointments, you can refer to the decision balance with the patient.

Exploring change	Reasons to drink (Cons)	Reasons to change (Pros)
Excess Alcohol Use	*1. Benefits* Enjoy drinking with my buddies Makes me feel relaxed Relieves stress Helps relieve back pain	*2. Concerns* Hangovers Spouse nags me High blood pressure Occasional stomach ache
Low-Risk Drinking or Abstinence	*3. Concerns* Miss my friends No fun Back-pain aggravation	*4. Benefits* Reduced risk of hypertension Spouse will be happy Less stomach upset
Force of change	Think score = 5 Feel score = 8	Think score = 5 Feel score = 2

The reason for inquiring about the benefits and concerns is to help patients think about factors that affect their resistance and motivation to change: in other words, their force of change toward disease or health. By working from the patients' perspective, you can enhance their cooperation to explore how alcohol is affecting their health, family, work, and other aspects of their life.

Once you have completed the decision balance, you can ask patients to score how important their reasons are to stay the same (resistance score) and to change (motivation score), using the questions below. Then, patients can monitor how their resistance and motivation scores change over time.

Explaining and Obtaining Resistance and Motivation Scores
"The left column represents your reasons to drink (resistance). The right column represents your reasons to cut down or quit drinking (motivation). On a scale of 0 to 10, 0 meaning none and 10 meaning very high, what score would you give for your reasons to stay the same? [pointing to the left column] *And what score would you give for your reasons to change? Are your resistance and motivation scores based on what you think or feel about change? Now how would you score your resistance and motivation based on what you* feel [if a think score was given] *or think [if a feeling score was given]?*

Decision balances can help patients think more about the possibility of change and clarify their ambivalence about change. The initial intent of using the decision balance is to itemize the benefits and concerns about drinking as usual versus low-risk drinking (or abstinence), without implying that patients should change. This approach can give you an insight into the reasons patients drink alcohol in spite of the associated risks and harms. The process itself is usually insufficient to initiate actual change in patients; it is only a first step in motivating them.

Use a decision balance with family members

If family members accompany the patient, you can ask them to do a decision balance separately from the patient. Afterwards, they can compare their perspectives. A family member's decision balance can help you and them understand why the patient and family members are at different stages of change. When a family member is at the action stage and the patient is at the contemplation stage about the patient's drinking habit, the family member may nag the patient to change (or be perceived as nagging) and evoke patient resistance. Thus, you can use the decision balance to help the patient and family members understand how they differ in their views about the benefits and concerns about change. This process can help family members understand the patient's resistance and ambivalence, but, more important, it can help them to stop nagging the patient.

At the end of the encounter, you can give the decision balances back to the patient and family members. Patients and family members can continue to work on this task by adding more items to their decision balance, and comparing the similarities and differences in their items. If they are willing, they can combine the items from both decision balances onto a new sheet of paper as part of an assignment for the next appointment.

Assess motivational reasons, competing priorities, energy and self-efficacy

Ask patients the reasons why they want to change. This inquiry can help you better understand whether patients are intrinsically or extrinsically motivated to change. You can also inquire about patients' energy and self-efficacy to change.

Assessing Motives
"Tell me what is driving you to consider changing your drinking habit." [Let the patient respond, and then continue with prompting.] *"Is it because of family and friends? Is it because you feel you ought to change? Are you doing it for yourself because it is important to you or perhaps for a combination of reasons? Which is most important?"*
Assessing Competing Priorities and Energy
"What competing priorities make it difficult for you to change your drinking habit?"   *"On a scale of zero to ten, how much energy can you put into changing your drinking habit?"*
Assessing Confidence and Ability (self-efficacy)
"On a scale of zero to ten, how would you rate your confidence to abstain from alcohol (for 2-4 weeks or for life)?"   *"On a scale of zero to ten, how would you rate your ability to abstain from alcohol (for 2-4 weeks or for life)?"*

Assess supports and barriers

Supports and barriers may facilitate or hinder patients' changing their drinking habits.

Assessing Supports
"Who is around to support you after you have quit drinking or kept to low-risk drinking? Do you feel that you want help from others to help you quit drinking or keep to low-risk drinking? Have you thought about attending AA meetings or getting an AA sponsor?"
Assessing Barriers
"Is there anyone who makes it more difficult for you to change your drinking habit? Are there any situations that make it difficult for you to cut down to low-risk limits or quit altogether for a while?"

B. Disease-centered Assessments

The options for a disease-centered assessment are listed in a sequence that ranges from less threatening to more threatening for the patient:

1. Discuss presenting complaints without addressing the patient's use of alcohol.
2. Link alcohol use to the presenting complaint.
3. Clarify the severity of hazardous, harmful, or dependent use of alcohol.

A disease-centered assessment also helps you define the severity of the alcohol problem. If patients are drinking above low-risk limits, then they are hazardous users of alcohol. Chapter 4a defined harmful and dependent use of alcohol and provided you with guidelines about using diagnostic uncertainty for negotiating with patients about making a specific diagnosis of excessive alcohol use. The language of these criteria has been modified into a questionnaire (Tables 4b.6 and 4b.7) that you can use with patients as a way to engage them in self-evaluation. You can use this questionnaire with patients during the encounter, or by patients alone after the encounter for future discussion. The information that patients provide can be used to educate them about their alcohol use. These questionnaires may also assist you in negotiating with patients about diagnosis. Patients can circle their responses (Y= Yes   Ns = Not sure   N = No).

Table 4b.6 Self-evaluation for Alcohol Problems	Circle One		
During the past year, have you had any problems caused by or made worse by alcohol use?			
1. Difficulties in fulfilling your responsibilities at work, school, or home	Y	Ns	N
2. Physical or mental health problems	Y	Ns	N
3. Repeated alcohol-related legal problems	Y	Ns	N
4. Social or relationship problems	Y	Ns	N

Table 4b.7 Self-evaluation for Alcohol Dependence	Circle One		
Spending more time drinking than on other activities:			
"Are you doing fewer other activities (social, occupational, or recreational)			
because you are more involved in drinking-related activities?"	Y	Ns	N
Spending more time obtaining alcohol and recovering from its effects:			
"Do you spend a fair amount of time in obtaining alcohol for your pleasure?"	Y	Ns	N
"Do you spend a fair amount of time recovering from the effects of alcohol?"	Y	Ns	N
Less able to control your alcohol use:			
"Do you have difficulty deciding when to stop drinking alcohol?"	Y	Ns	N
"Do you drink larger amounts of alcohol than you intended?"	Y	Ns	N
Urges and cravings to drink:			
"Do you have urges or cravings for alcohol?"	Y	Ns	N
Drinking despite its negative consequences:			
"Do you drink even though you know it causes you problems?"	Y	Ns	N
Development or loss of tolerance:			
"Do you need more alcohol than you used to in order to have the same effect?"	Y	Ns	N
"Can you drink much more alcohol than you used to before you get drunk?"	Y	Ns	N
"Do you need much less alcohol to have the same effect or to get drunk?"	Y	Ns	N
Withdrawal effects from alcohol:			
"Have you had any withdrawal effects when you stop drinking alcohol?"	Y	Ns	N
"Does drinking alcohol help relieve your withdrawal symptoms?"	Y	Ns	N

A response of "yes" to a question from three or more sections probably indicates physical or psychological dependence on alcohol.

STEP 4: ENHANCING MUTUAL UNDERSTANDING

Educate patients about your assessment and/or discuss further their self-evaluation about their alcohol use. This process may involve negotiating about the diagnosis (refer to Chapter 4a). After reaching some agreement about the problem, use nondirect and direct interventions, respectively, to lower resistance and enhance motivation to change. Also, consider whether to discuss how you and your patients view their self-efficacy, the same or differently.

A. Educate Patients about Excessive Alcohol Use

You can inform patients nonjudgmentally about the outcome of their assessment, so that they think more about the relationship of their alcohol use to their health concerns, and the likelihood of hazardous, harmful, or dependent use of alcohol. Such education also encourages patients to think more about the risks and harms, and, if relevant, the physical and psychological aspects, of addiction.

Alcohol use related to presenting complaint or health concerns: Address patients' presenting complaints but also educate them about how alcohol relates to their complaint.

Hazardous use: Inform patients that they are drinking beyond the low-risk limit[25] and then evaluate what they think about this information. Inform them about how their intake compares with that of the general population and how excessive use increases the risk of developing health care problems, particularly if they have a family history of alcoholism.

Harmful use: Educate patients about how alcohol is causing or contributing to medical, legal, social, sexual, psychological, and/or financial problems. Inform them about the need to assess further whether their alcohol use is causing any other health problems. Provide objective data about the medical consequences of drinking alcohol, such as the results of blood tests.

Alcohol dependence: Provide patients with assessment feedback about the level of dependence (e.g., tolerance, loss of control, and continued drinking despite negative consequences) and educate them about alcohol dependence.[26]

In the time-pressured environment of primary care and hospital settings, practitioners are often unable to make a comprehensive assessment of alcohol use in a single patient encounter, and consequently cannot make a definitive diagnosis. If necessary, in such situations you can present your assessment to patients in a tentative way (as described in Chapter 4a, page 65), and/or educate patients in personally meaningful ways that enable them to make their own diagnosis.

Counter patient resistance to diagnostic labeling

Even if you educate patients about their alcohol risk in nonjudgmental ways, some patients may respond defensively by stating that they are not an alcoholic or do not have a drinking problem.

Patient Defensiveness about Alcohol Dependence: *"You're not saying that I am an alcoholic, are you?"*
Practitioner's Response: *"What do you mean by 'an alcoholic'?"* [Reflective questioning]
   "That's a good question, but I don't know the answer. Together we can work out whether you are at risk of becoming one." [Validation with concern]

Patient: *"But I'm not a skid-row alcoholic."*
Practitioner's Response: *"Most alcoholics are not skid-row. Most have a job and an intact family. We no longer use the term 'alcoholic' for that reason. Instead, we use the term 'alcohol dependency.' Let me explain what this means."* [Reframing patient's definition]

Patient Defensiveness about Alcohol Abuse: *"Are you telling me that I have a drinking problem?"*
Practitioner's Response: *"I don't know about that, but it is important to find out whether alcohol is causing your health problems."* [Reframing the label]
   "Let me share with you the medical definition of a drinking problem—[alcohol abuse]—so that you can decide for yourself." [Clarifying differences]

Patient Defensiveness about Hazardous Use: *"I don't drink any more than my friends."*
Practitioner's Response: *"But you and your friends are in the minority. Most people don't drink as much as your friends do."* [Reeducating patient]

B. Use Nondirect Interventions to Lower Patient Resistance

It is equally important to know not only what to say but also how to say it when dealing with patients. A neutral stance helps you use nondirect interventions more effectively. In other words, you deliberately avoid trying to make patients change. At this stage, you do not state what is best for individual patients about whether, when, how, or why they should change. This nondirect exploration helps patients lower their resistance to change so that they become more inclined to consider it. Even if this does not occur, this approach is less likely to provoke patients to externalize their resistance so that they work against you. It is difficult, however, to maintain a stance of neutrality—not recommending what is best for individual patients—when you feel strongly that patients *should* change.

The different types of nondirect interventions are listed below, with specific examples that you can use or adapt for your own patients. These interventions are also discussed individually in the following section.

Nondirect Interventions to Lower Resistance
Use simple reflection to elicit ambivalence: *"So you like drinking when you go out?" "So drinking helps you to relax?" "So sometimes you get hangovers?"*
Probe priorities to explore ambivalence: *"What is the most important reason for you to drink? And what is the most important reason for you to change your drinking habit?"*
Use double-sided reflection to summarize ambivalence: *"On the one hand, drinking alcohol is fun, but, on the other hand, you get hangovers the following morning."*
Acknowledge ambivalence: *"So, it seems that you have mixed feelings about drinking alcohol."*
Emphasize personal responsibility and choice: *"What you decide to do about drinking is entirely up to you." "It's up to you to decide whether to change. I'm here only to see if you are interested in improving your health. That's what I see as my role. Only you can decide what is in your best interest."*
Use explore-the-future questioning: *"So, what do you think your health will be like in 5-10 years if you carry on drinking alcohol at the same or higher levels?"*

Use simple reflection to elicit ambivalence

By further exploring the benefits and concerns about drinking alcohol from patients' perspective, you may elicit some ambivalence from them about their alcohol use. Reflective statements ("So you like drinking with your buddies") encourage patients to elaborate on the statements made during the assessment when drawing up a decision balance.

Probe priorities to explore ambivalence

The purpose of exploring ambivalence is to clarify the key issues that patients are working on, and then to clarify the relative importance of these issues, as marked in each quadrant of the decision balance.

Use double-sided reflection to summarize ambivalence

Double-sided reflections can challenge patients to work through their ambivalence about change. Statements such as "On the one hand, you like to drink and party, but on the other hand, you are then less likely to practice safe sex" can clearly summarize a patient's ambivalence toward change. Patients need time, however, to reflect about such statements. Remaining silent after making such statements disrupts patients' automatic defensiveness, and gives them a timeout to reflect about inconsistencies in their rationalizations for engaging in risk behaviors.

Acknowledge ambivalence

Sometimes, it is worthwhile to acknowledge explicitly patients' ambivalence to change. This can help patients feel understood in ways that may keep them from feeling discouraged. You can help them to understand that this is part of the normal process when considering change.

Emphasize personal responsibility and choice

Emphasizing personal responsibility can serve several important functions for both you and your patients. For example, when you use nondirect interventions, some patients may interpret your intentions as implying that they should change. When this occurs, you can use variations of the examples described below to minimize patient resistance and help them feel they have a choice. This approach is also useful when you get "stuck," or when patients resist working with you for other reasons.

Use explore-the-future questioning

These types of questions helps patients to examine their past and present to explore the future in order to see the impact of their drinking habit. These questions can be modified to help patients explore their family history of drug and alcohol problems.

C. Use Direct Interventions to Motivate Patient Change

After patients become more receptive (less resistant) to the possibility of change, you can use direct interventions to enhance patient motivation to change. In effect, you act as an advocate for behavior change, but without telling patients what they should do. Direct interventions help patients alter their perceptions about the benefits and concerns about behavior change so that they diminish the value they give to reasons to stay the same, and increase the value they give to reasons to change. These interventions can help patients do most of the work, but resistance can occur particularly when they feel that you are trying to "make them change" their perceptions and values.

Use benefit substitution

You can ask patients how they could obtain the benefits of drinking in alternative ways. This task can be part of the patient encounter, or patients can complete this task for the next encounter or on their own time. After they have worked on developing their own ideas, you may add your suggestions. Again, let the patient do the work first before providing assistance.

Benefit Substitution
"What are other ways of having fun with your friends that don't involve drinking alcohol?" Or, *"You say that you enjoy drinking beer with your friends, but can you still enjoy your friends and drink non-alcoholic beer at lunchtime?"*

Use back-to-the-future questions

Back-to-the-future questions help patients anticipate the possibility of future complications or events (negative or positive) occurring in the present. These questions help patients consider what they would do if such a complication or event did occur.

Back-to-the-future
"If you were to develop a health problem from your drinking now, would you stop drinking?" [Provided that the patient shows some interest in prevention, continue.] *"At the moment, you are drinking over the low-risk drink limit and are at risk for developing complications. Do you want to wait and see if you develop a complication before deciding to change?"* [If the patient remains interested in prevention, continue.] *"What would it take for you to decide to drink alcohol below the low-risk limit?"* [If the patient is ambivalent, or not interested in prevention, continue.] *"Would you mind sharing with me why you don't want to avoid complications?"* Or, *"Let's suppose that alcohol is damaging your health in a way you are unaware of. Do you think this is a possibility?"* [With a negative response, offer an example such as abnormal liver function enzymes. With an affirmative answer, continue by saying:] *"If we discover that alcohol is damaging your health, what do you think you will do?"*

Clarify values

Interventions that probe and contrast patients' values may help them think about their life priorities in ways that go beyond what they itemized on their decision balance: for example, how alcohol use rates in relationship to other aspects of their life. A probing question involves asking patients to reflect about what is more important in their life than alcohol use. A contrasting question asks patients to compare whether alcohol (or drug) use is more important to them than something or somebody else, such as their relationship to their spouse, children, and/or grandchildren. Value clarification questions can be effective in focusing patients who are evasive, avoid responsibility for themselves, and/or blame others.

Clarifying Values
Questions that probe values: *"What is more important in your life than drinking alcohol?"* *"What is more important in your life than your health?"* *"What would have to change to make your health more important than drinking alcohol?"*
Questions that contrast values: *"So, having a hangover is worth it to have a good time at the party?"* *"So what is more important to you: drinking alcohol or having a good relationship with your spouse and being a good parent?"* *"You say that your wife is worried about your having a drinking problem, but you don't think you do. So what is more important to you: drinking alcohol, or having a wife who is less worried?"*
Questions that contrast values and behavior: *"If you say that your relationship with your wife is more important than drinking alcohol, you're saying one thing and doing another. What would convince you to do what you say?"*

Probing and Contrasting Values—Mrs. C. used cocaine once a month or so for several years when meeting with a group of friends to drink rum. MP asked: "Do you know of any people who have run into serious trouble with their use of cocaine?" [MP was indirectly attempting to ascertain whether Mrs. C. had any concerns about cocaine use, and whether she valued keeping out of trouble.] He then asked: "Do you think there's any possibility that this might happen to you?" [MP used a back-to-the-future question.] "Are there other things in your life that are more important to you than drinking alcohol and using cocaine?" [MP directly challenged the patient to think about how important cocaine use was compared to other things in her life.] MP then asked Mrs. C. about any concerns about cocaine use. Mrs. C. said, "I am concerned about avoiding sex with HIV-infected cocaine users, preserving my health, and avoiding addiction and financial bankruptcy."

Commentary: This approach placed the responsibility on Mrs. C. to reflect and clarify what was more important in her life than using alcohol and cocaine.

Challenge rationalizations

Patients often provide intriguing rationalizations for their excessive use of alcohol. From the patients' frame of reference, their rationalizations make reasonable or even indisputable sense, but to you, their rationalizations are irrational and flawed. Nondirect interventions help you understand patients' frames of reference. Direct interventions help you challenge patients' frames of reference in ways that may modify or change their rationalizations.

Challenging Rationalizations

"Do you mind if I say a few things that might help you think about your drinking differently?" [With an affirmative response from the patient, continue.] *"It may make you pause and think. You don't have to say anything if you don't feel like it, and if you want me to stop talking about alcohol, just tell me."* [Choose one of the following statements.] *"Many drinkers with family histories of alcoholism don't remember how many years it took for their father (or other family member) to become an alcoholic, so they believe that it is impossible for them to become an alcoholic like their father (or other family member)." "Sensible drinkers can even become alcoholics without knowing it: for example, they don't recognize how much they have developed a tolerance for alcohol."*

Examples of Responding to Rationalizations—Mr. D. (age 50) held two jobs to earn enough money to support his family. His second job was as a barman; he regarded this job as recreational, a release from work and family responsibilities. Mr. D. drank well over the low-risk drinking limit. During his encounter with his practitioner, he made a number of comments rationalizing his drinking habit. Dr. M. did not agree with Mr. D., and challenged him.

Patient: *"I never lose control when I drink alcohol and drive."*
Practitioner (challenging the patient's frame of reference): *"That is what most people think, but alcohol impairs people's judgment so that they think they are still in control. Alcohol affects your ability to drive without your being aware of it."*

Patient: *"I got a DWI but I wasn't drinking out of control."*

Practitioner: *"You may not feel out of control, but that's not the problem. Research shows that you may be able to do routine driving when you drink, but your reaction time and skills in emergency situations are impaired."*[27]

Patient: *"I am a sensible drinker."*

Practitioner: *"But you can still damage your health even if you are a sensible drinker."*

Patient: *"I hold down two jobs without any difficulty."*

Practitioner: *"You hold down two jobs very well, but that doesn't have much to do with how alcohol is affecting your health."*

Use discrepancies

During the process of understanding patients' reasons for drinking alcohol, you may identify discrepancies between their behaviors and some aspect of their self-interest, or help them discover these discrepancies for themselves.

Discrepancies between a Behavior and Self-interest
"You enjoy drinking alcohol at parties, but you get a hangover the morning after." "You say that alcohol makes you feel better. But if you felt better, would you still need to drink?"   *"I'm not sure if I'm hearing you correctly, but what I think I hear is that your relationship with alcohol is becoming more important than your relationship with your spouse and kids."*   *"You started drinking at home since your DWI, but now you're trapped at home with a wife who nags you about your drinking."*   *"You say that alcohol helps you with your depression. At best, alcohol gives you short-term relief by numbing your feeling of depression, but afterwards you'll feel worse because alcohol makes you more depressed. So you drink more. It becomes a vicious cycle. If alcohol really helped depression, you could stop using it after a while because your depression would go away. What do you think is the best way for you to treat your depression?"*   *"So, now that your kids are getting into alcohol and drugs, you're beginning to take another look at your own use of alcohol. How does their use of alcohol and drugs affect you and your thinking about your alcohol use?"*   *"You say that alcohol helps you sleep better, but the effects of this drug are complex. Let me explain. Alcohol certainly does help you get to sleep, but it also causes wakefulness during the night. This reduces the amount of deep sleep that your body needs to give you more energy. When asleep, you do not realize that your sleep is poor quality. So, in the evening, when you feel tired and have difficulty getting to sleep, you understandably have a few drinks to help you sleep. Do you understand what I'm saying? [Let the patient respond.] It is a kind of vicious cycle. What makes this worse is that when your body has become accustomed to the alcohol, you experience worse sleep problems when you stop drinking because of the rebound effect. It may take a week or so, sometimes longer, for your body to get over the effects of alcohol. It is quite complicated to understand how alcohol affects sleep. What do you think is the best way for you to improve your quality of sleep and regain your energy, so that you feel better?"*

Learning Exercise 4b.1: Drug substitute request

In response to practitioners pointing out such discrepancies, patients may request a drug substitute instead of alcohol. Take a minute to reflect about how you would respond to these requests, and fill in your responses below.

Request for a Drug	Your Response
"I can't possibly stop drinking alcohol unless I have something to help me sleep. Can you give some Valium to take at night?"	
"You just don't understand my difficulties—the sleeping problem and the stresses that I am under. I really need something at night to help me sleep."	
"There must be some safe pill you could give me to help me sleep."	

Reframe items, issues, and events

Reframing techniques help patients to change their views about items, issues, or events related to their decision balance. In other words, you help patients turn a reason to drink into a reason not to drink, enhance a reason to stop/reduce drinking alcohol, and/or diminish a reason to drink.

Reframing Items, Issues, or Events
Change a reason to drink into a reason not to drink: *"You can certainly hold your liquor, but drinking so much alcohol puts you at an increased risk for developing cirrhosis and becoming an alcoholic."*
Enhance a reason to stop/reduce drinking alcohol: *"You say that your spouse nags you about your drinking, but this shows how much your spouse is really concerned about your health. Are you willing to reduce your drinking to stop the nagging?"*
Diminish a reason to drink: *"You say that alcohol helps you get to sleep, but drinking alcohol decreases the quality of your sleep, which then makes you feel tired all the time."*

Use amplified reflection

You may identify issues, feelings, concerns, or lack of concern, and then reflect them back to the patient in an amplified form. For example, a patient mentioned that his father had cirrhosis of the liver, which was probably the cause of his death. He mentioned this without expressing any concern about the fact that his practitioner had just told him that he drank above low-risk limits and had elevated liver enzymes.

Challenging Claims or Positions Using Amplified Reflection
"So, alcohol makes you feel really happy." "So, alcohol makes your pain completely go away." "So, drinking alcohol is the best way for you to have fun with your friends." "So, your [wife/husband] is completely unjustified in [her/his] concerns about your drinking." "Your drinking is increasing your liver enzymes and increasing your risk of developing cirrhosis. Yet when you mentioned that your father died of cirrhosis..." [Pause. Let the patient respond and, assuming an indifferent, nonverbal response, then continue.] *"Yet you don't seem at all concerned about what I've just told you."* [Amplified reflection of the patient's nonverbal response]

Use differences in motivational reasons

Identify something other than alcohol use that patients are highly motivated to do (be a good parent or spouse, do well at work, fish for relaxation). Ask them if they could put the same amount of effort and care into changing their alcohol intake as they are putting into these other activities. Or, identify a past successful change (e.g., quitting smoking) and ask them to use that experience to help them change their alcohol use.

Using Differences in Motivational Reasons
"You decided to quit smoking by yourself, but what would it take for you to do the same thing in terms of reducing your alcohol intake to below low-risk limits?"

Monitor changes in resistance and motivation scores

Patients are ready for change when they, not you, perceive the reasons to change (motivation) as outweighing the reasons not to change (resistance).[28] To monitor change over time, you can ask patients if they have changed their resistance and motivation scores and why. Their explanations for changing their scores provide invaluable information about why things are getting better or worse, over time.

Monitoring Changes in Resistance and Motivation Scores
"What scores would you now give for your resistance and motivation to change, on a scale of 0-10? Why did you change your resistance score? And why did you change your motivation score? You can learn a lot about yourself even if your scores got worse and went in the wrong direction. Sometimes it helps if your resistance score goes up and your motivation score goes down, as it can show you what it would take to change for good."

D. Clarify Differences in Perceptions about Patient Self-efficacy

Patients may overestimate or underestimate their self-efficacy (ability and confidence) to change. Some patients who are unknowingly dependent on alcohol may even boast about their ability to quit drinking and also refute any need to change because their drinking is not causing any problems. In contrast, you may know that a particular patient is dependent on alcohol, and that alcohol is causing problems for the patient. To address this discrepancy in perception about self-efficacy, you can pose hypothetical statements:

"Suppose you were to accept a challenge—say, quit drinking for two weeks—to prove that you could do it without difficulty. What would you think if you discovered that you could not stop drinking and that you were dependent on alcohol without knowing it?"

On the other hand, some patients underestimate their self-efficacy to change their behavior. You can clearly state how you perceive their abilities to change differently, as a way to boost their confidence, and help them realistically reevaluate their strengths.

"On a scale of zero to ten, you stated that your ability to stop drinking was a 'one,' but I see you as a five to six on that scale. What do you think about the fact that we see things differently?"

(See Chapter 11b in *Beyond Advice: Becoming a Motivational Practitioner* for other ways to help patients deal with their sense of hopelessness about change.)

STEP 5: IMPLEMENTING A PLAN FOR CHANGE

The extent to which you and your patients share similar and different perceptions about the benefits, risks, and harms of alcohol use influences how you develop an appropriate plan together. If you underestimate the differences in these perceptions, you are likely to experience more difficulties in implementing a plan with your patients.

Clarifying Persistent Differences in Perceptions
"I think it is important for us to be clear about how we each see the benefits, risks, and harm of drinking alcohol—the same or differently—because this will affect how we work together. I think I understand what you like about drinking alcohol, but I am more concerned about the risks and harm caused by your drinking than you are. What do you think?"

A. Evaluate Patient Commitment toward a Plan

Before selecting goals for change and implementing a plan, consider assessing the extent to which patients are committed to changing their use of alcohol with respect to competing priorities, energy, and motivational reasons.

Competing Priorities
"What is going on in your life that makes it difficult for you to reduce your alcohol intake to low-risk levels (or to abstain) now? Is there anything else?" "What would it take for you to put low-risk drinking (or abstinence) at the top of your list of things to do?" "What is stopping you from putting low-risk drinking (or abstinence) at the top of your list of things to do?"
Energy
"What's going on that makes it difficult for you to devote your energy to quit drinking or cut down on your drinking? What would it take for you to put your energy into changing your drinking habit? If you don't have any energy to change, what would it take for you to get your energy back?"
Motives
"What will make you commit yourself to the goal of low-risk drinking (or abstinence)? And what else?" "You say that you are here because your family wanted you to come. But what would it take for you to come for your own reasons?"

B. Decide about Goals for Change

You need to decide for yourself what you think are the best goals for change based on your understanding of your patients, their readiness to change and the severity of their alcohol risk. The range of goals for implementing a plan may exist along the following continua: stages of change (contemplation-preparation-action), short-term/long-term goals, and pragmatic/ideal recommendations.

Range of goals

Table 4b.9 outlines a range of goals for helping hazardous, harmful and dependent drinkers. These options are:

- Contemplate further low-risk drinking or abstinence
- Prepare for low-risk drinking or abstinence
- Take action toward change (low-risk drinking or abstinence)

With regard to abstaining, drinking below low-risk limits, or reducing their alcohol intake and the duration for these goals, patients may opt for goals that are short-term (2-4 weeks) or long-term (greater than a year). When patients are unsure about the need for change or are ambivalent about it, they may opt for short-term, incremental steps toward change, such as reducing alcohol intake. If patients are reluctant to change, you can suggest that patients conduct an experiment and try to abstain for two weeks.

Before selecting goals, decide what your recommendations are going to be for the patient: either to abstain from alcohol, or to drink below the low-risk limits. Your opinion and recommendations will influence whether you think that you can work with this patient, or whether you will need to make a referral to an addiction specialist or a community program such as Alcoholics Anonymous.

Table 4b.8: Range of Goals for Changing Hazardous and Harmful Use of Alcohol

Think more about:
    Reduced alcohol intake, low-risk drinking, and abstinence.
    Use a decision balance to consider these goals.
Prepare for change:
    Plan how to deal with change.
    Learn about what constitutes alcohol abuse and dependence.
    Inform family and friends about plans to change.
Set a date to change (abstinence, low-risk, or reduced use):
    Short-term (2-4 weeks) vs. long-term goal.
    Address alcohol-related problems.

Treatment Options for Alcohol Dependence

Referral to a counselor for an in-depth assessment
Detoxification (outpatient vs. inpatient)
Referral to an alcohol program (outpatient vs. inpatient)
Attend Alcoholics Anonymous meetings
    • Attend open meetings
    • Get a sponsor
    • Attend 12-step, closed meetings
Use of Naltrexone to prevent relapse [29]

Setting goals

You can influence the goal-setting process by providing advice in either a disease-centered or patient-centered way, or by using a negotiated approach.

Practitioner-centered goal-setting:

Authoritarian (controlling) monologue— *"I think you should stop drinking alcohol altogether so that you don't get cirrhosis."*

Authoritative and autonomy-supportive monologue— *"If you continue to drink, you are at increased risk of developing cirrhosis. If you decide to stop drinking, you won't get cirrhosis."*

Patient-initiated goal-setting:

Advice-giving monologue— *"You seemed concerned when we talked about your father developing cirrhosis. Let me just mention something that you may have already thought about. Given the fact that your liver function tests are abnormal, you are also at risk of developing cirrhosis. Fortunately, the condition is reversible if you do something about it. Now, let me explain. If you were to stop drinking for six weeks, we could check your liver enzymes after that time to see whether they returned to normal."*

If an advice-giving approach does not work, negotiate with patients about whether to change.

Negotiated Approach—An Engaging Dialogue

MP: *"I am concerned because your father developed cirrhosis, and your blood test is now showing that your liver enzymes are high."*

Mr. W.: *"What does that mean?"*

MP : *"Let me explain. I think the amount of alcohol that you drink is causing some liver damage and putting you at increased risk of developing cirrhosis."* MP spoke in a low-key way and caring tone of voice. He showed the patient the written report of the test and explained what the results meant.

Mr. W.: *"I can't believe what you are telling me. I know that I don't drink as much as my father did."* Mr. W. paused, as if expecting the practitioner to reply. MP deliberately remained silent to let Mr. W reflect about this information. *"Is there something that I can do to stop this?"*

MP: *"Before we talk about that, let me explain a little something about your dad. Your father probably did not know that his liver tests were abnormal before he started drinking heavily. Had someone told him, he may have changed his drinking habits before developing cirrhosis."* MP again used silence to allow the patient to reflect about what he had said.

Mr. W: *"What are you telling me—to stop drinking?"* Mr. W. asked in an incredulous tone of voice.

Practitioner: *"I think you need to decide what is in the best interest of your health. Only you can decide whether you are prepared to do something about the abnormal liver tests and reduce your risk of developing cirrhosis."* MP respected Mr. W.'s autonomy to decide what to do about his health.

Mr. W: *"How do you know whether things will get better if I stop drinking? I mean, will I have to stop drinking for life?"*

MP: *"Fortunately, the liver enzyme levels can go back to normal. Let me share with you what I think you can do to check out if this will happen. If you were to stop drinking for six weeks, we could recheck the liver enzymes then to find out whether they return to normal. I don't know the answer yet to your second question. Let's first check out whether the liver damage is reversible or not. Time will help us work out whether it is necessary for you to stop drinking completely to avoid developing cirrhosis over time."* MP noticed that he was overwhelming the patient emotionally and deferred giving any further information. *"What do you think about what I'm telling you?"*

Mr. W: *"I think I should give up drinking for a while,"* Mr. W. said, but not as if he were convinced. *"Do you agree?"*

MP deliberately avoided answering that question: *"I am quite willing to tell you what I think you should do. But it is important for me to know what you can do to improve your own health. I am willing to help you in whatever you want."*

Mr. W.: *"I am still interested in what you think I should do."* Mr. W. now demonstrated a genuine interest in his practitioner's recommendations.

MP: *"Are you willing to stop drinking over the next six weeks to see whether your liver enzymes go back to normal?"* MP carefully posed his recommendation as a question rather than a statement.

Mr. W.: *"I am willing to try, but I think that I'll need a sleeping pill because alcohol helps me sleep."*

Requests for drugs

In response to motivational interventions, patients may reply in ways that challenge you to deal with requests for drugs. With a trial of abstinence, patients may feel that they need to substitute a drug for alcohol to help them deal with depression, anxiety, and/or difficulties in sleeping. A learning exercise will help you think about how to respond to such requests.

Learning Exercise 4b.2: Responding to the patient's request for sleeping tablets

Imagine that you are the practitioner. After reading the following dialogue, how would you respond to this patient?

Patient: *"I need a sleeping pill. Why don't you give me some diazepam?"*

Practitioner: *"So your sleeping problem is so bad that you are willing to substitute one drug for another. Do you see any alternative to using drugs?"*

Patient: *"Maybe later. Right now, if you don't give me something to sleep I can't possibly stop drinking alcohol. I have too much stress going on. I need something now!"*

Practitioner: *"Do you have so much stress that you are willing to risk using another drug, even though it is not dealing with the cause of the problem?"*

Patient *(after a period of silence):* *"Well, I suppose that's right."*

Practitioner: *"Can I tell you about how diazepam and alcohol affect your sleep?"*

Patient: *"Well, okay."*

Practitioner: *"Diazepam and alcohol may help in the short run, but not in the long run."* [This is agreement with a twist: contrasting short-term benefits with long-term concerns.] *"The effects of diazepam wear off in the short run, and then you need to increase the dose to help you sleep. When this happens, you can become addicted to it."* [The educational message focuses on concerns about use.] *"Do you understand why I am concerned about using drugs to deal with sleep problems?"*

Patient: *"Well, I guess so. But I really need something for a few weeks to help me sleep. Is there anything else I could use that is not addictive?"*

Practitioner: *"You just told me something that is really important."* [Again, the practitioner intervenes to help the patient identify a discrepancy and uses silence to foster self-reflection.]

Patient (after a moment of silence): *"You just don't understand my sleeping problem and the stresses that I am under. If you had my stresses, you would understand my sleeping problem better. There must be a safe pill you can give me. Can't you think of anything else?"*

Practitioner: [The practitioner noticed that the patient had shifted the agenda, but refocused on exploring whether the intervention had had any impact.] *"A moment ago, I noticed that you were silent. Do you mind if I ask you what was going through your mind?"* [This intervention invites the patient to put aside his defensive routines against considering change.]

Patient: *"I was thinking that I had better not become like my father."*

Think about whether you would use a drug with this patient before reading on.

Dealing with a request for sedative drugs

Patient: *"You just don't understand my sleeping problem and the stresses that I am under. If you had my stresses, you would understand my sleeping problem better. There must be a safe pill that you can give me. Can't you think of anything else?"*

Practitioner: *"Well, there are other drugs, such as amitriptyline, that are not addictive. You use this drug for a few weeks until your sleep problem settles down. But you can't take this drug with alcohol. Would you be prepared to stop drinking if you use this drug?"*

Patient: *"I need something to help me sleep."*

Practitioner: *"Amitriptyline often causes a dry mouth in the morning, but it wears off over time."*

Patient: *"What happens if the drug does not work?"*

Practitioner: *"We can talk over the phone about increasing the dose. But are you prepared to stop drinking?"*

Patient: *"Yes, I will."*

Practitioner: *"I'll start you off with a prescription for 25 mg a day and increase by one tablet every two to three days, up to three tablets a day. If you develop any other side effects besides dry mouth, call me and I will call you back. How soon can you come back to see me?"*

Patient: *"I could make it next Thursday afternoon."*

Some practitioners would never prescribe amitriptyline for several reasons—substituting one drug for another, for example, or concerns about drug interactions. In contrast, other practitioners may selectively use this drug in certain circumstances. To consider this issue, you can use a decision balance to explore the advantages and disadvantages of prescribing this drug versus never using it.

Set a date for change

You can help patients set a date to change based on whatever their goals are: thinking about change, preparing for change, attempting a trial of abstinence or low-risk drinking for 2-4 weeks, or aiming for the long-term goal of abstinence or low-risk drinking.

C. Work toward Solutions

You can use the MED-STAT solution-based approach to help patients evaluate the feasibility of achieving their goals for change.[30]

Interventions	Solution-based Approach
Miracle question (explore change)	*"Suppose a miracle happened tomorrow and you stopped drinking (or kept to low-risk drinking). What would your life be like then? How do you think your family and friends would respond?"*
Exceptions (identify strengths)	*"What was going on at times when you drank less alcohol compared to times when you drank more alcohol?* [Patient responds that he drinks when he gets angry.] *What happens on those occasions when you get angry and don't drink alcohol?"*
Difference (use strengths)	*"What can you learn from those occasions when you were angry and didn't drink alcohol?"* [Let the patient respond.] *"How can that help you deal with your anger when you are tempted to drink?"*
Scaling (assess motivation, self-efficacy and outcome expectancy)	*"On a scale of zero to ten, how would you rate your (motivation, ability and confidence) not to drink when you get angry? How would you rate whether you can achieve your goal for change (outcome expectancy)? What would increase or decrease your scores? Can you make a list of these reasons? Was there a time when your scores were higher than now? What would it take to tip the balance in favor of higher scores?"*
Timeouts (consider alternatives)	*"What other ideas do you have about how you could handle your anger differently instead of drinking alcohol?"* [Probe silences.] *"A moment ago, I asked you a question and you were silently thinking. What was going on?"*
Accolades (enhance efficacy)	*"You have the skills to keep to low-risk drinking (or abstain), but what would it take for you keep using your skills all the time?"*
Task appraisals (encourage action)	*"How do you know whether low-risk drinking or abstinence is the best goal for you?"*

STEP 6: FOLLOWING THROUGH

A. Rationale, Purpose, and Reasons for Follow-up

The rationale for recommending follow-up appointments has to be grounded in your experience with a patient, after you have worked through the problem-solving phases of enhancing mutual understanding and implementing a plan. At one extreme, you may develop a rationale for focusing on a particular alcohol-related problem (e.g., indigestion) without making it explicit that you will explore how alcohol affects indigestion at the next appointment. The rationale given to the patient may not entirely reflect your purpose for the next appointment. This "go-slow" approach may seem deceptive, but it is helpful when you anticipate that you are dealing with resistant patients who do not think that they have a drinking problem. At the other extreme, alcohol-dependent patients who accept their diagnosis may only need an explanation about the need for detoxification and immediate referral. After providing your rationale for a follow-up appointment, clarify with the patient about his or her reasons for making a follow-up appointment. This may help you understand the extent to which you have a common agreement about the reason for a follow-up.

Rationale for Follow-up Appointment
"I think it's important for you to come back and work out [choose one or more of the following]: *"What's causing your indigestion (or any other alcohol-related harm)."* *"Whether there's a relationship between your alcohol use and your indigestion."* *"Whether to decrease your alcohol intake so it doesn't bother your indigestion as much."* *"Whether you might be developing a drinking problem."* *"Whether you're becoming dependent on alcohol."* [Then arrange a follow-up appointment.]
Clarifying Patients' Reasons to Attend a Follow-up Appointment
"Why is it important for you to attend a follow-up appointment?" *"What do you think is the most important reason for you to attend a follow-up appointment?"* *"What health concerns do you want to address at your next appointment? When do you think will be a good time for you to come back and address your health concerns? You can always call me if you have any concerns about how the medication is working, or if you have any concern about side effects."*

B. Timing, Duration and Frequency of a Follow-up Appointment

Once you have established the rationale for a follow-up appointment, you can ask patients when they would like to come back and see you and how often. You may not always have the time to negotiate about arranging a follow-up appointment, but an example is provided next.

MP asked Mrs. D. when she thought she needed to come back for a follow-up appointment. Mrs. D was taken aback and asked, "When do you think?" MP explained that he was very interested in hearing first about what she thought before saying what he thought. She was surprised by this request. She paused and said, "I don't know." MP remained silent to allow her to reflect. Mrs. D. then asked, "What about four weeks?" MP then had two options: to accept Mrs. D.'s offer or to negotiate about a different time for the follow-up appointment if there was a large discrepancy between his opinion and Mrs. D.'s suggestion.

Timing, Duration and Frequency of Follow-up Appointment
"When do you think you should come back to see me?" *"When do you think it would be a good time for you to come back to check up on your health concerns?"* *"I think it's important for you to decide how often you should come back for a follow-up appointment. I will certainly share what I think about this, but I'm more interested in what you think."*

C. Methods to Ensure Change and Prevent Relapse
1. A diary to track change

When patients are contemplating changing their drinking habits, you can suggest that they keep a drinking diary as a way to help prepare them for change. Over a one-week period, you can ask patients to keep a record of the times and circumstances under which they drank alcohol, and to monitor their urges and what triggered their desire to drink. You can also use drinking diaries as a way to monitor progress toward the goal of low-risk drinking or abstinence.

A Diary for Tracking Change
"Are you willing to keep a drinking diary and write down your thoughts and feelings about your successes and difficulties in working toward your goal?"

2. Relapse prevention

As part of relapse prevention, ask patients to monitor their temptations, urges, and cravings to drink alcohol. In addition, you can warn patients that positive or negative emotions (feeling happy, bad, guilty, anxious, depressed) are common triggers for relapse, and ask them how they will handle these emotions in alternative ways. You can also help coach them on strategies to anticipate high-risk situations.

Relapse Prevention
Management of risk situations: *"What kind of situations will make it difficult for you to keep to your goal of low-risk drinking or abstinence? In what ways can you deal with those situations?"*
Pharmacologic management: *"Have you encountered any difficulties in taking your Naltrexone on a regular basis? Do you have any concerns about taking the medication?"*
Emotional management: *"When you feel that way (any negative emotions), how do you think you can deal with those feelings instead of drinking alcohol?"*
Reevaluation of supports: *"Would it help to have someone who will help you work toward your goal for abstinence (or low-risk drinking)?"*
Reevaluation of barriers: *"What do you think is making it difficult for you to abstain or keep to low-risk drinking limits? How do you think you're going to handle those situations?"*
Use of positive reinforcement: *"Would it be helpful for you to set up a reward for abstaining or keeping to low-risk drinking limits? What would that be?"*

3. Motivational reevaluation

Ask patients to use their decision balance to reevaluate and/or reinforce the need for preventing lapses or relapses.

Motivational Reevaluation
"Let's look again at your decision balance and talk about whether you still think that your reasons to change are really more important than your reasons to stay the same. This may help you stick to low-risk drinking or abstinence when you feel that you could lapse or relapse."

MOVING ON

This chapter provided a broad range of options that you can use with patients who drink excessive amounts of alcohol. In some instances, you may provide brief advice to hazardous drinkers, who may decide to change as a consequence of a three-minute intervention. In other instances, it may take multiple encounters, or even several years, before you can help a patient confront his or her alcohol dependence and accept a referral to a counselor for assessment and/or treatment. The next chapter adapts this same approach to address smoking cessation.

Reference List

1. Miller WR, Baca LM. Two-year follow-up of bibliotherapy and therapist-directed controlled drinking training for problem drinkers. Behavior Therapy 1983;14: 441-448
2. Miller WR, Sovereign RG. The check-up: A model for early intervention in addictive behaviors. In: Loberg T, Miller WR, Nathan PE, et al., eds. Addictive behaviors: Prevention and early intervention. Amsterdam: Swets & Zeitlinger; 1989:219-231
3. Valle SK. Interpersonal functioning of alcoholism counselors and treatment outcome. Journal of Studies on Alcohol 1981;42: 783-790
4. Luborsky L, McLellan AT, Woody GE, et al. Therapist success and its determinants. Arch Gen Psych 1985;42: 602-611
5. Bradley KA, Bush KR, McDonell MB, et al. Screening for problem drinking: comparison of CAGE and AUDIT. Ambulatory Care Quality Improvement Project (ACQUIP). Alcohol Use Disorders Identification Test. J Gen Intern Med 1998;13: 379-388
6. Wallace PG, Brennan PJ, Haines AP. Drinking patterns in general practice patients. Journal of the Royal College of General Practitioners 1987;37: 354-357
7. Rydon P, Redman S, Sanson-Fisher RW, et al. Detection of alcohol-related problems in general practice. Journal of Studies on Alcohol 1992;53(3): 197-202
8. Lawner K, Doot M, Gausas J, et al. Implementation of CAGE alcohol screening in a primary care practice. Fam Med 1997;29: 332-335
9. Lairson DR, Harrist R, Martin DW, et al. Screening for patients with alcohol problems: severity of patients identified by the CAGE. J Drug Educ 1992;22: 337-352
10. Ewing JA. Detecting alcoholism. The CAGE questionnaire. JAMA 1984;252: 1905-1907
11. Buchsbaum DG, Buchanan RG, Centor RM, et al. Screening for alcohol abuse using CAGE scores and likelihood ratios. Annals of Internal Medicine 1991;115: 774-777
12. Saunders JB, Aasland OG, Babor TF, et al. Development of the Alcohol Use Disorders Identification Test (AUDIT): WHO Collaborative Project on Early Detection of Persons with Harmful Alcohol Consumption—II. Addiction 1993;88(6): 791-804
13. Allen JP, Litten RZ, Fertig JB, et al. A review of research on the Alcohol Use Disorders Identification Test (AUDIT). Alcohol Clin Exp Res 1997;21: 613-619
14. Piccinelli M, Tessari E, Bortolomasi M, et al. Efficacy of the alcohol use disorders identification test as a screening tool for hazardous alcohol intake and related disorders in primary care: a validity study. BMJ 1997;314: 420-424

15. Bush K, Kivlahan DR, McDonell MB, et al. The AUDIT alcohol consumption questions (AUDIT-C): an effective brief screening test for problem drinking. Ambulatory Care Quality Improvement Project (ACQUIP). Alcohol Use Disorders Identification Test. Arch Intern Med 1998;158: 1789-1795

16. Piccinelli M, Tessari E, Bortolomasi M, et al. Efficacy of the alcohol use disorders identification test as a screening tool for hazardous alcohol intake and related disorders in primary care: A validity study. British Medical Journal 1997;314: 420-424

17. Seppa K, Lepisto J, Sillanaukee P. Five-shot questionnaire on heavy drinking. Alcohol Clin Exp Res 1998;22: 1788-1791

18. Aertgerts B, Buntinx F, Ansoms S, et al. Screening properties of questionnaires and laboratory tests for the detection of alcohol abuse or dependence in a general practice population. British Journal of General Practice 2001;51: 206-217

19. Brown RL, Leonard T, Saunders LA, et al. A two-item screen test for alcohol and other drug problems. The Journal of Family Practice 1997;44: 151-160

20. Schorling JB, Willems JP, Klas PT. Identifying problem drinkers: Lack of sensitivity of the two-question drinking test. American Journal of Medicine 1995;98: 232-236

21. Taj N, Devera-Sales A, Vinson DC. Screening for problem drinking: Does a single question work? The Journal of Family Practice 1998;46: 328-335

22. Dawson DA, Archer LD. Relative frequency of heavy drinking and the risk of alcohol dependence. Addiction 1993;88: 1509-1518

23. Dawson DA. Consumption indicators of alcohol dependence. Addiction 1994;89: 345-350

24. Ferguson RA, Goldberg DM. Genetic markers of alcohol abuse. Clinica Chimica Acta 1997;257: 199-250

25. Klatsky AL. Annotation: Alcohol and longevity. American Journal of Public Health 1995;85: 16-18

26. National Institute on Alcohol Abuse and Alcoholism. Alcohol and tolerance. Alcohol Alert 1995;28: 1-4

27. National Institute on Alcohol Abuse and Alcoholism. Drinking and driving. Alcohol Alert 1996;31

28. Prochaska JO, DiClemente CC, Norcross JC. In search of how people change: Applications to addictive behaviors. American Psychologist 1992;47(9): 1102-1114

29. Weinrieb RM, O'Brien CP. Naltrexone in the treatment of alcoholism. Annual Review of Medicine 1997;48: 477-487

30. Giorlando ME, Schilling RJ. On becoming a solution-focused physician: The MED-STAT acronym. Families, Systems & Health 1997;15: 361-373

CHAPTER 5a

TOBACCO USE

FOR REFLECTION

How can you combine behavioral interventions with drug treatment of nicotine dependence to help your patients quit their tobacco use?

OVERVIEW

Traditional approaches to tobacco cessation involve practitioners providing education and advice to patients.[1-5] These approaches, however, help only a small percentage of tobacco users (2%-10%) to quit each year.[6,7] Factors that enhance quit rates include the intensity and duration of smoking cessation programs, and approaches that use multiple methods rather than single methods. For example, drug treatments for nicotine dependence can complement behavioral treatments and thus enhance quit rates among nicotine-dependent smokers. The key issue is how best to combine behavioral interventions with treatments for nicotine dependence to help smokers quit.

TOBACCO USE

Tobacco is the single greatest preventable contributor to disease and premature death internationally, causing 4 million deaths a year. Adolescent and adult smoking is increasing in most parts of the world. Within 20-30 years, tobacco use will cause 10 million deaths per year, accounting for one in eight deaths overall; 70% of all these deaths will occur in developing countries.[8] The report "Trust Us: We're the Tobacco Industry" helps to understand how the tobacco industry contributed toward creating this pandemic plague.[a] To counteract these disease-promoting practices, the World Health Organization has sponsored a Tobacco-free Initiative to decrease global tobacco consumption (http://www.who.int/toh/).

Internationally, a number of evidence-based reviews, guidelines and reports have been published about the need to address tobacco use and to treat tobacco dependence.[9-19] Additional information about tobacco cessation and control are available on Web sites listed in Tables 5a.6-5a.9. A summary of the recent Agency for Healthcare Research and Quality (AHRQ) Guideline on Treating Tobacco Use and Dependence highlights key issues and findings[20] (the full report is downloadable from www.ahrq.gov/guide).

1. Tobacco dependence is a chronic condition that often requires repeated interventions to enhance quit rates and permanent abstinence.
2. Effective tobacco dependence treatments are available for patients who are willing to quit.

- Treatments involving person-to-person contact (or by individual, group, or pro-active telephone counseling) are consistently effective, and their effectiveness increases with treatment intensity (e.g., minutes of contact).
- Three types of counseling and behavioral therapies (problem solving/skills training, intra-treatment social support, and extra-treatment social support) were found to be especially effective and should be used for all patients attempting tobacco cessation.
- In the absence of contraindications, all tobacco users should be offered drug treatments for their quit attempts. First-line options include nicotine replacement therapies (gum, inhaler, nasal spray, or patch) and bupropion SR. Second-line options include clonidine and nortriptyline. For patients not ready to quit, motivational interventions can help them think about quitting and work toward a quit attempt in the future.

---

a. You can download the full report (html) from www.ash.org.uk/html/conduct/html/trustus.html, or the pdf format from http://tobaccofreekids.org/campaign/global/framework/docs/TrustUs.pdf

3. Tobacco dependence treatments are both clinically effective and cost effective. Health care systems should reimburse practitioners for tobacco counseling and pharmacological treatment of nicotine dependence.

4. Health care systems must develop the organizational infrastructure support in health care settings, so that they can systematically identify all tobacco users and monitor the impact of treatment on patients over time.

Booklets for consumers, clinicians, health care administrators, and insurers/purchasers accompany this guideline:

- *You Can Quit Smoking; Helping Smokers Quit* (consumer guide)
- *A Guide for Primary Care Clinicians. Smoking Cessation: Information for Specialists. Quick Reference Guide*
- *Smoking Cessation: A Systems Approach*
- *A Guide for Health Care Administrators, Insurance, Managed Care Organizations and Purchasers*

The economic implications of tobacco use on health are enormous.[21;22] Furthermore, the treatment of nicotine dependence is cost effective: $3,539 per life-year saved.[23;24] In contrast, the cost of 3-vessel coronary bypass graft surgery (vs. medical management) is $12,000 per life-year saved, and the cost of the same surgery for mild and severe angina (vs. percutaneous coronary angioplasty) is $23,000 and $100,000 per life-year saved, respectively.[25] In spite of the far superior cost effectiveness of prevention, greater emphasis is still placed on treating tobacco-related diseases.

KEY FINDINGS

The data about cessation interventions generate conflicting interpretations. These commentaries range from pessimistic and realistic to optimistic. Pessimistic commentaries make the following conclusions:

- One behavioral intervention for smoking cessation is no better than another in the clinical context.[26;27]
- Behavioral interventions are of limited effectiveness.[28-30]
- A meta-analysis concluded that behavioral interventions are not cost effective.[31]
- Multimodal behavioral therapy actually averaged 2% greater reductions in smoking cessation, compared to the control groups. Little progress has been made in enhancing the smoking cessation rates over the past 40 years.[32]

Optimistic commentaries highlight studies on brief counseling that show higher quit rates (25%) than those for advice (5%-10%).[33] Intensive treatments for outpatients and hospital inpatients have achieved long-term success rates ranging from 15%-25%.[5;34] Smokers with cardiorespiratory complications may have higher quit rates when they receive personalized interventions.[35-40]

AHRQ Intervention Data

Meta-analyses from the AHRQ guideline provide the most comprehensive and up-to-date information about interventions for tobacco cessation. This data is summarized in Tables 5a.1-5a.5. The percentage of attributable benefit is the impact that the intervention had over no treatment or a control group. The number needed to treat (NNT) is the number of patients that need to be treated to produce one favorable outcome. For more details about confidence intervals and references, consult the full publication.

Table 5a.1: Impact of Screening System for Tobacco Users in Health Care Settings on Clinical Intervention and Abstinence Rates

Assessing Impact of No Screening versus Screening System on:	Comparing % rates	% Attributable Benefit (95% CI)	Number Need to Treat
A. Clinical intervention rate	38.5 vs. 65.6	27.1 (19.8, 34.1)	4
B. Abstinence rate	3.1 vs 6.4	3.3 (-1.8, 8.5)	30

Clearly, screening systems for tobacco users are essential organizational supports for maintaining higher rates of interventions and for achieving higher abstinence rates.

Table 5a.2: Impact of Clinical Interventions on Tobacco Abstinence Rates

Assessing Impact of:	Comparing % rates	% Attributable Benefit (95% CI)	Number Need to Treat
No advice vs. physician advice	7.9 vs. 10.2	2.3 (0.4, 4.1)	43
No contact vs. < 3-minute session	10.9 vs. 13.4	2.5 (0.0, 5.2)	40
vs. 3- to 10-minute session	vs. 16.0	5.1 (1.9, 8.3)	20
vs. >10-minute session	vs. 22.1	11.2 (8.5, 13.8)	9
0-1 session vs. 2-3 sessions	12.4 vs. 16.3	3.9 (1.3, 6.6)	26
vs. 4-8 sessions	vs. 20.9	8.5 (5.7, 11.2)	12
vs. > 8 sessions	vs. 24.7	12.3 (8.6, 16.0)	8
No clinician vs. self-help	10.2 vs. 10.9	0.7 (-1.1, 2.5)	143
vs. nonphysician	vs. 15.8	5.6 (2.6, 8.6)	18
vs. physician	vs. 19.9	9.7 (3.5, 16.0)	10
No clinician vs. 1 clinician	10.8 vs. 18.3	7.5 (4.6, 10.3)	13
vs. 2 clinicians	vs. 23.6	12.8 (12.8, 17.9)	8
vs. > 3 clinicians	vs. 23.0	12.2 (9.2, 15.1)	8

Table 5a.3: Impact of Different Methods on Tobacco Abstinence Rates

Assessing Impact of No format vs.:	Comparing % rates	% Attributable Benefit (95% CI)	Number Need to Treat
Self-help	10.8 vs. 12.3	1.5 (0.1, 2.8)	67
Proactive telephone counseling	vs. 13.1	2.3 (0.6, 4.0)	43
Group counseling	vs. 13.9	3.1 (0.8, 5.3)	32
Individual counseling	vs. 16.8	6.0 (3.9, 8.3)	17
One format	10.8 vs. 15.1	4.3 (2.0, 6.6)	23
Two format	vs. 18.5	7.7 (5.0, 10.3)	13
Three format	vs. 23.2	12.4 (9.1, 15.8)	8
One type of self-help	14.3 vs. 14.4	0.1 (-1.4, 1.6)	1000
Two or more types of self-help	vs. 15.7	1.4 (-2.0, 4.9)	71

Overall, a multimodal, multimethod and interdisciplinary approach is clearly more effective than relying on one single intervention or discipline.

Table 5a.4: Impact of Behavioral Methods on Tobacco Abstinence Rates

Assessing Impact of No Counseling vs.:	Comparing % rates	% Attributable Benefit (95% CI)	Number Need to Treat
Intra-treatment social support	11.2 vs. 14.4	3.2 (1.1, 5.3)	31
Extra-treatment support	vs. 16.2	5.0 (0.6, 9.4)	20
General problem solving	vs. 16.2	5.0 (2.8, 7.3)	20
Other aversive smoking	vs. 17.7	6.5 (0.0, 13.7)	15
Rapid smoking	vs. 19.9	8.7 (0.0, 17.8)	11

The treatment labels for these behavioral methods are non-specific and include a variety of interventions. The AHRQ guideline does not address the interactive effects of using different behavioral methods. As a complement to these behavioral methods, vigorous exercise was found to boost quit rates in women.[41]

SPECIFIC ISSUES

A number of factors increase and decrease the prospects of long-term abstinence of tobacco use. Tobacco users who are motivated to quit, ready to quit within a month period, confident in their ability to quit, and/or have a social supportive network are more likely to achieve long-term abstinence. Conversely, tobacco users with high nicotine dependence, a history of psychiatric comorbidity, and high stress levels are less likely to achieve long-term abstinence.

Behavioral interventions are an integral part of tobacco cessation programs. In addition, most patients need some assistance in overcoming their nicotine dependence. The 5As model, as outlined in the AHRQ guideline, can be summarized as:

1. Ask about tobacco use
2. Advise to quit
3. Assess willingness to quit
4. Assist in quit attempt
5. Arrange follow-up

This basic, practical model is a good initial step, but the guideline does not provide practitioners with adequate guidance in how to help patients at follow-up visits, nor how to engage patients in the change process who are not ready to quit. Chapter 5b presents how practitioners can learn ways of addressing these clinical challenges.

A. Drug Treatment of Nicotine Dependence

High levels of nicotine dependence enhance the difficulty of quitting.[42;43] Heavy smokers are half as likely to quit smoking with self-help interventions than are lighter smokers.[44] Withdrawal symptoms may cause a relapse rate of 25%-60%; patients relapse most frequently within the first six months (particularly within the first few days or weeks) after quitting.[45] You can use the Fagerström Tolerance Questionnaire (see Table 5a.10, page 119) to estimate the degree of nicotine dependence of your patients.[44;46] Clinically, you can estimate an increased risk for relapse if patients:

- Have had marked withdrawal symptoms on previous quit attempts
- Smoke more than 25 cigarettes a day
- Have difficulty refraining from smoking in restricted areas
- Smoke more in the morning
- Smoke their first cigarette soon after waking (within 30 minutes)
- Smoke when bedridden with illness
- Inhale more deeply[47-49]

The typical smoker absorbs about 1-3 mg of nicotine per cigarette, totaling 20-40 mg for each pack per day. To avert significant withdrawal symptoms, patients need at least 50% of their usual amount of nicotine. Nicotine replacement therapy (NRT) improved treatment outcome.[32;44;46;49-57] A meta-analysis of the benefits of nicotine replacement therapy concluded that the patch and chewing gum increased smoking cessation rates 9% and 6% respectively, compared to controls.[58] NRT has uncertain efficacy in primary care, however, when only minimal behavioral support is provided.[59]

Drug treatment of nicotine dependency helps to ease the withdrawal symptoms and to enhance tobacco cessation rates.[60] A comparison of the impact of different drug treatments for nicotine treatment is summarized in Table 5a.5, page 113.

Table 5a.5: Impact of Pharmacotherapy on Tobacco Abstinence Rates

Assessing Impact Placebo vs.	Comparing % rates	% Attributable Benefit (95% CI)	Number Need to Treat
Nicotine gum	17.1 vs. 23.7	6.6 (3.5, 9.6)	15
Nicotine inhaler	10.5 vs. 22.8	12.3 (5.9, 18.7)	8
Nicotine spray	13.9 vs. 30.5	16.6 (7.9, 25.3)	6
Nicotine patch	10.0 vs. 17.7	7.7 (6.0, 9.5)	13
Over-the-counter patch*	6.7 vs. 11.8	5.1 (0.8, 4.2)	20
One NRT vs two NRTs	17.4 vs. 28.6	11.2 (4.3, 18.0)	9
Bupropion SR	17.3 vs. 30.5	13.2 (5.9, 20.5)	8
Second-line treatment options			
Clonidine	13.9 vs. 25.6	11.7 (3.8, 19.7)	9
Noritriptyline	11.7 vs. 30.1	18.4 (6.4, 29.9)	5

*This data is from one study only [61]

NRT cardiovascular risks and drug dependency

The nicotine patch does not increase the rate of acute cardiovascular events[62-64] even in patients who smoke on the patch.[65] The Lung Health study on chronic obstructive pulmonary disease, however, found that 38% of women and 30% of men were still using nicotine gum at 12 months.[66] With free access to nicotine gum, 15% to 20% of successful abstainers will continue to come for a year or longer.[67] NRT is much less harmful than tobacco use.[68]

Pharmacological treatment of tobacco use in pregnancy

Pregnant smokers should be encouraged to quit first without pharmacological treatment. Drug treatments may be used in pregnancy and during lactation, if the benefits of tobacco abstinence outweigh the risk of treatment and continued tobacco use. The FDA classification for using these drugs in pregnancy are listed below: Class A (controlled studies demonstrate remote risk) through Class D (some human fetal risk, but the benefits must outweigh the risks), and Class X (drugs are contraindicated in pregnancy).

Class A	None identified yet
Class B	Bupropion SR
Class C	Nicotine patch, clonidine
Class D	Nicotine gum/inhaler/spray, noritriptyline*

*Noritriptyline has been associated with a few case reports of possible limb reduction anomalies.

Nicotine gum

Nicotine gum improves the smoking cessation rate by approximately 40%-60%, compared to control groups at a year follow-up. The dose of the nicotine gum is 2 or 4 mg, of which 50% is absorbed through the mouth. The higher dose gum is more effective with highly dependent smokers. Patients slowly chew the gum until they notice a tingling sensation or peppery taste in the mouth, and then place the gum between the cheek and gums. After this sensation resolves, patients can start chewing again and go through the same cycle. Chewing too fast can release nicotine rapidly and cause side effects: mouth soreness, hiccups, dyspepsia, and jaw ache. The gum can be used up to 12 weeks, with no more than 24 pieces per day. As a guideline, patients can chew a piece of gum every 1-2 hours for the first six weeks, every 2 to 4 hours for the next three weeks, and then every 4-8 hours for the next three weeks. Adherence to appropriate gum usage is associated with higher smoking cessation rates.[26]

Nicotine inhaler

Patients can take 6-16 inhalations per day for up to six months, with the goal of gradually decreasing the number of inhalations per day over several weeks.[69;70] Each inhalation delivers 4 mg of nicotine. Side effects include mouth and throat irritation (40%), coughing (32%), and rhinitis (32%); these symptoms declined with continued use. Patients should avoid drinking and eating 15 minutes before and after each inhalation. The inhaler has the advantage of giving quitters a substitute for the hand-to-mouth behavior of smoking. This method is most similar to the gum, as the inhaler delivers nicotine into the mouth whether or not the patient inhales deeply. In cold weather (below 40°F), patients need to know that the inhaler does not work well.

Nicotine patch

These patches come in different dose regimens according to the manufacturer's specifications. The duration of treatment is usually eight weeks, with gradual decrements in the dose regimen every 2-6 weeks (refer to Web sites listed in Table 5a.9). Treatment of longer than eight weeks does not improve the quit rate; 16- and 24-hour patches work equally as well. Patients may experience mild irritation at the application site of the patch and dizziness as side effects. The patches at least doubled the success rate of other behavioral therapies.[71;72 72] Half of all users developed local skin reactions. Rotating patch sites and use of topical steroids (1% hydrocortisone cream) may reduce these reactions, but 5% of patients discontinue the patch due to the skin reaction.

Nicotine spray

With their head tilted slightly back, patients can spray 0.5 mg of nicotine into each nostril, but without inhaling it. They can use 1 to 2 doses per hour (a minimum of 8 and a maximum of 40 doses per day) for 3-6 months. Users (94%) report moderate to severe nasal irritation in the first two days which reduces in severity, but 84% still report some irritation after three weeks. The nasal spray method delivers nicotine more quickly than the gum, patch, or inhaler, but less rapidly than cigarettes. This may explain why 15%-20% of patients use the spray for more than six months, and 5% used the spray at higher doses than recommended.

Bupropion SR

Bupropion decreases a person's urge to smoke and is effective in helping nondepressed smokers to quit.[73] In a double-blind controlled trial, the rates of smoking cessation at seven weeks were 19.0% in the placebo group, 28.8% in the 100 mg group, 38.6% in the 150 mg group, and 44.2% in the 300 mg group (p<0.001). At one year, the respective rates were 12.4%, 19.6%, 22.9%, and 23.1%. The rates for the 150 mg group (p=0.02) and the 300 mg group (p=0.01) —but not the 100 mg group (p=0.09) —were significantly better than those for the placebo group.[74]

Clonidine

The FDA has not yet approved clonidine for smoking cessation, but it appears an effective treatment. A clear dose-response has not been established. The dose range used in trial is 0.15-0.75 mg per day, or 0.1-.0.2 mg/day transdermally (TTS). This initial dose is 0.1 mg twice a day, or 0.1 mg TTS, increasing by 0.1 mg per week, if needed. Treatment may be continued for 3 to 10 weeks. Side effects include: dry mouth (40%), drowsiness (33%), constipation (10%), sedation (10%; caution is needed while driving and using machinery), and reduced blood pressure that needs monitoring. Rebound hypertension, agitation, confusion and tremor may occur if this drug is not stopped after 2-4 days.

Noritriptyline

The FDA has not yet approved noritriptyline for smoking cessation, but it appears an effective treatment. The initial dose is 25 mg per day, increasing gradually to 75-100 mg for up to 12 weeks. This treatment should be started 10-28 days before the quit date. Side effects include: sedation (caution is needed while driving and using machinery), dry mouth (64%-78%), lightheadness (49%), shaky hands (23%), blurred vision (16%), and urinary retention. Noritriptyline should be used with caution in cardiovascular disease and in patients at risk for suicide because of its toxicity and overdose effects in causing arrythmias.

Pharmacological and behavioral interventions

A question exists whether brief advice improves the outcome of NRT.[26:27] Better outcomes are achieved when nicotine gum is combined with intensive behavioral treatment.[59] Patients, however, use less gum in primary care than in clinic-based programs.[75] The difference in success rates between primary care and clinic-based programs may relate to the improved adherence to NRT rather than the independent effect of behavioral interventions.[26] Such an interpretation of this data only heightens the need to develop more effective behavioral interventions that have an additive or synergistic effect on the beneficial impact of NRT.

B. The Need for Innovation, Improvisation and Integration

As previously noted, the analysis of the smoking cessation data provides a spectrum of different commentaries that span the pessimistic-optimistic continuum.

Meta-analyses provide information on aggregate performance about smoking interventions but do not inform you about best practices. Published articles and guidelines do not provide enough information to understand what makes up the different categories of behavioral interventions. Furthermore, these different behavioral methods contain multiple interventions, so it becomes increasingly difficult to identify which aspects of these interventions work best for a particular patient. Thus, guidelines cannot inform you about which are the best practices for particular situations or which specific interventions are best for individual patients.

The AHRQ guideline presents the results of these meta-analyses in isolation from one another, consonant with the reductionistic, scientific method. In contrast, tobacco cessation programs must be integrated into complex systems of health care delivery. Furthermore, these programs must use multi-modal, multi-method and interdisciplinary approaches in ways that have additive and synergistic effects on organizations, practitioners and patients. Health care settings must implement and improve complex interventions over time and monitor their impact on helping patients change over time. These interventions need to address both the organizational processes of implementing tobacco cessation programs but also enhance the potency of behavioral interventions that work in additive or synergistic ways with the drug treatment of nicotine dependence. In other words, health care systems and settings must innovate, improvise, and monitor the impact of using both organizational and behavioral interventions well beyond the duration of randomized controlled trials. No guideline can provide hard evidence on how to do this.

The AHRQ smoking guideline predominantly emphasizes the use of the 5As model: a brief health education and advice approach. The guideline also describes a motivational approach to smoking cessation in terms of risks, relevance, rewards, and repetition, but without giving sufficient details about how to implement this approach into practice.[7] The Smokescreen program is another example of such a motivational approach that attempts to enhance patients' readiness to quit smoking.[76] Such an approach to smoking cessation is appropriate when advice-giving approaches do not work.[77] But these approaches are not well developed in terms of helping patients move from not thinking about quitting to thinking about it. Chapter 5b addresses this issue, and the Web site www.MotivateHealthyHabits.com has a videostreamed demonstration in how to do this.

MOVING ON

This chapter highlighted the need to use pharmacological treatments of nicotine dependence. Chapter 5b describes how you can develop individualized interventions for resistant, indifferent, and ambivalent smokers and enhance their readiness to change over time. The innovative and synergistic use of pharmacological and behavioral interventions will determine the future success of tobacco cessation programs.

Table 5a.6: Web Sites for Addressing Tobacco Control and Cessation

Organization	Web or E-mail Address
WHO Tobacco-free Initiative	www.who.int/toh/
Framework for Tobacco Control	www.fctc.org
International Non-Governmental Coalition	www.ingcat.org
International Newsletter on Tobacco	http://lists.essential.org/mailman/listinfo/intl-tobacco
International Agency on Tobacco and Health	admin@iath.org
International Union Against Cancer (UICC)	www.uicc.org
Prevention of Tobacco Induced Diseases	www.ptid.org
Global Partners for Tobacco Control	www.essentialaction.org/
Tobacco Control: An International Journal	www.tobaccocontrol.com
WHO (Europe) and SRNT	www.treatobacco.net/
European Network of Women Against Tobacco	margaretha.haglund@fhinst.se
GLOBALink	www.globalink.org
Cochrane database	www.cochranelibrary.com/
UK Report on smoking in England	www.doh.gov.uk/public/smoking.htm
UK Report on preventing youth smoking	www.york.ac.uk/inst/crd/ehcb.htm
Health Development Agency	www.hea.org.uk
Cochrane Tobacco Addiction Group	lindsay.stead@dphpc.ox.ac.uk
ASH (Action on Smoking and Health)	www.ash.org.uk
U.S. Surgeon General on Tobacco Use	www.surgeongeneral.com/ and search tobacco
U.S. Surgeon General on Tobacco Use in Women	www.surgeongeneral.gov/library/womenandtobacco/
CDC's Office on Smoking and Health	www.cdc.gov.tobacco
CDC's How to Quit	www.cdc.gov/tobacco/how2quit.htm
CDC's Tobacco Information & Prevention Source	www.cdc.gov/tobacco/index.htm
CDC's Comprehensive Tobacco Control Programs	www.cdc.gov/tobacco/bestprac.htm
CDC's Tobacco Research, Data and Reports	www.cdc.gov/tobacco/data.htm
CDC's School Health ProgramGuidelines	www.cdc.gov/nccdphp/dash/guide.htm
Agency for Health Care Research and Quality	www.ahrq.gov/guide
U.S. Office of Personnel Management	www.opm.gov/ehs/smokmod2.htm
American Lung Association	www.lungusa.org
Addressing Tobacco in Managed Care	www.aahp.org/atmc.htm
American Academy of Family Physicians	www.aafp.org
American Cancer Society	www.cancer.org
National Cancer Institute	www.nci.nih.gov
National Heart, Lung and Blood Institute	www.nhlbi.nih.gov/index.htm
Society for Research on Nicotine and Tobacco	www.srnt.org
Tobacco Control Resource Centre	www.tobacco-control.org
Advocacy Institute	www.scarcnet.org
American Medical Association (AMA)	www.ama-assn.org
Office on Smoking and Health	www.cdc.gov/nccdphp/osh/tobacco.htm
TobaccoWeek	www.tobaccowars.com/
The Truth	www.thetruth.com
Second Hand Smoke Resource	www.repace.com/factsheet.html
BADvertising	www.badvertising.org/

UK White Paper on Tobacco Use www.official-documents.co.uk/document/cm41/4177/4177.htm

Table 5a.7: Web Sites for Adult Smoking

Organization	Web Address
Quit smoking online	www.quitsmokingonline.com
You can quit	www.mnbluecrosstobacco.com/mndec/resources/youcanquit.html
You can quit consumer guide	www.surgeongeneral.gov/tobacco/consquits.htm
The last draw	www.thelastdraw.com
Online support for nicotine addiction	www.nicotine-anonymous.org/
Smoker Stoppers	www.smokestoppers.com/proga.dll/home.html
Quitnet – Quit all together	www.quitnet.org/qn_main.jtml
CNN interactive site on smoking	http://cnn.com/HEALTH/indepth.health/smoking/
Your online Smoking Advisor	www.stop-tabac.ch/
Wellness Web Smokers' Clinic	www.wellweb.com/smoking/SMHOMEP2.HTM#whatsnew
Well med	www.wellmed.com
Gordian Health Solutions	www.gordian-health.com
Health Media	www.healthmedia.com

Table 5a.8: Web Sites for Youth Smoking

Organization	Web Address
Tips for Teens	www.qweb.org/Ext/CDCTips.htm
Message to Youth	www.tobaccofree.org/children.html
Nicotine Free Kids	www.nicotinefreekids.com
Smoke Free Kids	www.smokefreekids.com
U Beat Their Butts	www.beatbutts.com
Campaign for Tobacco-Free Kids	www.tobaccofreekids.org
Teen Tobacco Chewing	www.patchproject.com

Community interventions for preventing youth smoking.
http://www.update-software.com/abstracts/ab001291.htm
Systematic reviews about health promoting U.K. schools and health promotion in schools (1999)
http://www.hta.nhsweb.nhs.uk/_vti_bin/shtml.dll/monodown.htm.

Table 5a.9: Web Sites about Treating Nicotine Dependence

Treatment Options	Web Address
Nicoderm patch	www.nicodermcq.com
Nicorette gum	www.nicorette.com
Nicotrol patch	www.nicotrol.com
Zyban	www.zyban.com

Table 5a.10: Fagerström Test[46]

Questions	Answers	Points
A. How soon after you wake do you smoke your first cigarette?	Within 5 minutes	3
	6-30 minutes	2
	31-60 minutes	1
	After 60 minutes	0
B. Do you find it difficult to refrain from smoking in places where it is forbidden, e.g., at the library, in church, at the theater?	Yes	1
	No	0
C. Which cigarette would you hate to give up most?	First in a.m.	1
	All others	0
D. How many cigarettes a day do you smoke?	10 or less	0
	11-20	1
	21-30	2
	31 or more	3
E. Do you smoke more frequently during the first hours after waking than during the rest of the day?	Yes	1
	No	0
F. Do you smoke if you are so ill that you are in bed most of the day?	Yes	1
	No	0

Reproduced with permission

If you score four points or more on this test, you may very well be addicted to nicotine. Scores of more than six generally are interpreted as indicating a high degree of dependence, with a more severe withdrawal syndrome, greater difficulty in quitting, and possibly the need for higher doses of medication. The option of using nicotine replacement therapy (gum and/or patch and/or inhaler) to treat the withdrawal syndrome can complement and enhance the outcome of using behavioral approaches.

Reference List

1. American Academy of Family Physicians. AAFP Stop Smoking Program: Patient stop smoking guide. American Academy of Family Physicians; 1987

2. National Heart Lung and Blood Institute, American Association for Respiratory Care. How you can help patients stop smoking: Opportunities for respiratory care practitioners. U.S. Department of Health and Human Services; 1989

3. National Heart Lung and Blood Institute, The American Lung Association, and The American Thoracic Society. Clinical opportunities for smoking intervention: A guide for the busy physician [NIH Publication No. 92-2178]. 1992. Bethesda, MD, U.S. Department of Health and Human Services.

4. National Cancer Institute. How to help your patients stop smoking: A National Cancer Institute manual for physicians [NIH Publication No. 89-3064]. 1989. Bethesda, MD, National Institutes of Health.

5. Orleans CT, Glynn TJ, Manley MW, et al. Minimal-contact quit smoking strategies for medical settings. In: Orleans CT, Slade J, eds. Nicotine addiction: Principles and management. New York: Oxford University Press; 1993:181-220

6. Glynn TJ, Manley MW. How to help your patients stop smoking: A National Cancer Institute Manual for Physicians [NIH Publication No. 89-3064]. Bethesda, MD: U.S. Department of Health and Human Services; 1989

7. The Smoking Cessation Clinical Practice Guideline Panel and Staff. The Agency for Health Care Policy and Research *Smoking Cessation Clinical Practice Guideline* . JAMA 1996;275: 1270-1280

8. World Health Organization. Investing in health research and development. Geneva: World Health Organization; 1996

9. Tobacco Advisory Group, Royal College of Physicians. Nicotine Addiction in Britain. 2000. London, Royal College of Physicians.

10. Peto R, Lopez A. Future worldwide health effects of current smoking patterns. In: Koop CE, Pearson CE, Schwarz MR, eds. Critical Issues in Global Health. San Francisco: Jossey-Bass; 2000:

11. World Health Organization, Europe. Partnership to Reduce Tobacco Dependence. 2000. Copenhagen, World Health Organization.

12. West R, McNeill A, Raw M. Smoking cessation guidelines for health professionals: an update. Health Education Authority. Thorax 2000;55: 987-999

13. World Health Organization. Conclusions of conference on the regulation of tobacco dependence treatment products. 1999. Copenhagen, World Health Organization.

14. Lancaster T, Stead L, Silagy C, et al. Effectiveness of interventions to help people stop smoking: findings from the Cochrane Library [see comments]. BMJ 2000;321: 355-358

15. Agence National d'Accreditation et d'Evaluation en Sante. Consensus Conference on Smoking Cessation (English summary by Jacques Le Houezec). 1999. Paris, ANAES.

16. The Cochrane Collaboration. Cochrane Database of Systematic Reviews. 1999. The Cochrane Library.

17. British Thoracic Society. Smoking cessation guidelines and their cost-effectiveness. Thorax 1998;53: S1-S38

18. Department of Health and Human Services. The Health Consequences of Smoking: Nicotine Addiction: A Report of the Surgeon General. 88-8406. 1988. Atlanta, US Department of Health and Human Services. Public Health Service, Centers for Disease Control, Center for Chronic Disease Prevention and Health Promotion. Office of Smoking and Health. DHHS Publication No. (PHS) (CDC) 88-8406.

19. American Medical Association. American Medical Association guidelines for the diagnosis and treatment of nicotine dependence: how to help patients stop smoking. 1994. Washington, D.C., American Medical Association

20. Fiore MC, Bailey WC, Cohen SJ, et al. Treating Tobacco Use and Dependence. Clinical Practice Guideline 2000;343: 1772-1777

21. World Bank. Curbing the Epidemic. Governments and the Economics of Tobacco Control. 1999. Washington, World Bank

22. Manning WG, Keeler EB, Newhouse JP, et al. The costs of poor health habits. Cambridge, MA: Harvard University Press; 1991

23. Parrott S, Godfrey C, Raw M, et al. Guidance for commissioners on the cost effectiveness of smoking cessation interventions. Health Educational Authority. Thorax 1998;53 Suppl 5 Pt 2: S1-38

24. Cromwell J, Bartosch WJ, Fiore MC, et al. Cost-effectiveness of the clinical practice recommendations in the AHCPR guideline for smoking cessation. JAMA 1997;278: 1759-1766

25. Wong JB, Sonnenberg FA, Salem DN, et al. Myocardial revascularization for chronic stable angina: Analysis of the role of percutaneous transluminal coronary angioplasty based on data available in 1989. Annals of Internal Medicine 1990;113: 852-871

26. Lichtenstein E, Glasgow RE. Smoking cessation: what have we learned over the past decade? J Consult Clin Psychol 1992;60: 518-527

27. Hajek P. Current issues in behavioral and pharmacological approaches to smoking cessation. Addictive Behaviors 1996;21: 699-707

28. Raw M. The treatment of cigarette dependence. In: Israel Y, Glaser FB, Kalant H, et al., eds. Research advances in alcohol and drug problems, vol. 4. New York: Plenum Press; 1978:441-485

29. Lichtenstein E. The smoking problem: A behavioral perspective. Journal of Consulting & Clinical Psychology 1982;50: 804-819

30. Jarvis M. Helping smokers give up. In: Pearce S, Wardle J, eds. The practice of behavioral medicine. London: BPS Books; 1989:284-305

31. Law M, Tang JL. An analysis of the effectiveness of interventions intended to help people stop smoking. Archives of Internal Medicine 1995;155: 1933-1941

32. Shiffman S. Smoking cessation treatment: any progress? J Consult Clin Psychol 1993;61: 718-722

33. Glynn TJ. Relative effectiveness of physician-initiated smoking cessation programs. Cancer Bulletin 1988;40: 359-364

34. Orleans CT. Treating nicotine dependence in medical settings: A stepped-care model. In: Orleans CT, Slade J, eds. Nicotine addiction: Principles and management. New York: Oxford University Press; 1993:145-161

35. Richmond RL, Webster IW. A smoking cessation programme for use in general practice. Medical Journal of Australia 1985;142: 190-194

36. Windsor RA, Cutter G, Morris J, et al. The effectiveness of smoking cessation methods for smokers in public health maternity clinics: A randomized trial. American Journal of Public Health 1985;75: 1389-1392

37. Risser NL, Belcher DW. Adding spirometry, carbon monoxide, and pulmonary symptom results to smoking cessation counseling: A randomized trial. Journal of General Internal Medicine 1990;5: 16-22

38. Fisher EB, Jr., Haire-Joshu D, Morgan GD, et al. Smoking and smoking cessation. American Review of Respiratory Disease 1990;142: 702-720

39. Ockene J, Kristeller JL, Goldberg R, et al. Smoking cessation and severity of disease: The Coronary Artery Smoking Intervention Study. Health Psychology 1992;11: 119-126

40. Gritz ER, Kristeller J, Burns DM. Treating nicotine addiction in high-risk groups and patients with medical co-morbity. In: Orleans CT, Slade J, eds. Nicotine addiction: Principles and management. New York: Oxford University Press; 1993:279-309

41. Marcus BH, Albrecht AE, King TK, et al. The efficacy of exercise as an aid for smoking cessation in women: a randomized controlled trial [see comments]. Arch Intern Med 1999;159: 1229-1234

42. Shiffman S. Tobacco "chippers": Individual differences in tobacco dependence. Psychopharmacology 1989;97: 539-547

43. Pinto RP, Abrams DB, Monti PM, et al. Nicotine dependence and likelihood of quitting smoking. Addictive Behaviors 1987;12: 371-374

44. Pomerleau CS, Pomerleau OF, Majchrzak MJ, et al. Relationship between nicotine tolerance questionnaire scores and plasma cotinine. Addictive Behaviors 1990;15: 73-80

45. Brandon TH, Tiffany ST, Obremski KM, et al. Postcessation cigarette use: the process of relapse. Addict Behav 1990;15: 105-114

46. Heatherton TF, Kozlowski LT, Frecker RC, et al. The Fagerstrom Test for Nicotine Dependence: A revision of the Fagerstrom Tolerance Questionnaire. British Journal of Addiction 1991;86(9): 1119-1127

47. Hughes JR, Hatsukami DK, Pickens RW, et al. Consistency of the tobacco withdrawal syndrome. Addictive Behaviors 1984;9: 409-412

48. Fagerstrom KO. Effects of nicotine chewing gum and follow-up appointments in physician-based smoking cessation. Preventive Medicine 1984;13: 517-527

49. Killen JD, Fortmann SP, Telch MJ. Are heavy smokers different from light smokers? A comparison after 48 hours without cigarettes. JAMA 1988;260: 1581-1585

50. Killen JD, Fortmann SP. Role of nicotine dependence in smoking relapse: Results from a prospective study using population-based recruitment methodology. International Journal of Behavioral Medicine 1994;1: 320-334

51. Hughes JR. Combined psychological and nicotine gum treatment for smoking: A critical review. Journal of Substance Abuse 1991;3: 337-350

52. Fagerstrom KO, Schneider NG. Measuring nicotine dependence: A review of the Fagerstrom Tolerance Questionnaire. Journal of Behavioral Medicine 1989;12: 159-182

53. Abrams DB, Follick MJ, Biener L, et al. Saliva cotinine as a measure of smoking status in field settings. American Journal of Public Health 1987;77: 846-848

54. Niaura R, Goldstein M, Abrams D. A bioinformational systems perspective on tobacco dependence. British Journal of Addiction 1991;86: 593-597

55. Pomerleau OF, Collins AC, Shiffman S, et al. Why some people smoke and others do not: New perspectives. Journal of Consulting & Clinical Psychology 1993;61: 723-731

56. Killen JD, Fortmann SP, Kraemer HC, et al. Who will relapse? Symptoms of nicotine dependence predict long- term relapse after smoking cessation. Journal of Consulting & Clinical Psychology 1992;60: 797-801

57. Pomerleau OF, Rosecrans J. Neuroregulatory effects of nicotine. Psychoneuroendocrinology 1989;14: 407-423

58. Tang JL, Law M, Wald N. How effective is nicotine replacement therapy in helping people to stop smoking? BMJ 1994;308: 21-26

59. Lam W, Sze PC, Sacks HS, et al. Meta-analysis of randomised controlled trials of nicotine chewing gum. Lancet 1987;2: 27-30

60. Fiore MC, Jorenby DE, Baker TB, et al. Tobacco dependence and the nicotine patch. Clinical Guidelines for effective care. JAMA 1992;268: 2687-2694

61. Leischow SJ, Muramoto ML, Cook G, et al. OTC nicotine patches: effectiveness alone and with brief physician intervention. American Journal of Health Behavior 1999;23: 61-69

62. Benowitz NL, Gourlay SG. Cardiovascular toxicity of nicotine: implications for nicotine replacement therapy. J Am Coll Cardiol 1997;29: 1422-1431

63. Joseph AM, Norman SM, Ferry LH, et al. The safety of transdermal nicotine as an aid to smoking cessation in patients with cardiac disease. N Engl J Med 1996;335: 1792-1798

64. Mahmarian JJ, Moye LA, Nasser GA, et al. Nicotine patch therapy in smoking cessation reduces the extent of exercise-induced myocardial ischemia. J Am Coll Cardiol 1997;30: 125-130

65. Working Group for the Study of Transdermal Nicotine in Patients with Coronary Artery Disease. Nicotine replacement therapy for patients with coronary artery disease. Archives of Internal Medicine 1994;154: 989-995

66. Nides MA, Rakos RF, Gonzales D, et al. Predictors of initial smoking cessation and relapse through the first 2 years of the Lung Health Study. Journal of Consulting & Clinical Psychology 1995;63: 60-69

67. Hajek P, Jackson P, Belcher M. Long-term use of nicotine chewing gum. Occurrence, determinants, and effect on weight gain. JAMA 1988;260: 1593-1596

68. Henningfield JE. Nicotine medications for smoking cessation. N Engl J Med 1995;333: 1196-1203

69. Hjalmarson A, Franzon M, Westin A, et al. Effect of nicotine nasal spray on smoking cessation. Archives of Internal Medicine 1994;154: 2567-2572

70. Sutherland G, Stapleton JA, Russell MAH, et al. Randomised controlled trial of nasal nicotine spray in smoking cessation. Lancet 1992;340: 324-329

71. Fiore MC, Smith SS, Jorenby DE, et al. The effectiveness of the nicotine patch for smoking cessation: A meta-analysis. JAMA 1994;271: 1940-1947

72. Silagy C, Mant D, Fowler G, et al. Meta-analysis on efficacy of nicotine replacement therapies in smoking cessation. Lancet 1994;343: 139-142

73. Benowitz NL. Treating tobacco addiction—nicotine or no nicotine? New England Journal of Medicine 1997;337: 1230-1231

74. Hurt RD, Sachs DP, Glover ED, et al. A comparison of sustained-release bupropion and placebo for smoking cessation [see comments]. N Engl J Med 1997;337: 1195-1202

75. Jackson PH, Stapleton JA, Russell MA, et al. Nicotine gum use and outcome in a general practitioner intervention against smoking. Addictive Behaviors 1989;14: 335-341

76. Richmond R. Educating medical students about tobacco: Teachers' manual and students' handouts. In: Richmond R, ed. Educating medical students about tobacco: Planning and implementation. Paris, France: Tobacco Prevention Section, Int. Union Against Tuberculosis and Lung Diseases; 1996:15-59

77. Botelho RJ. When "quit smoking" advice doesn't work: Use motivational approaches. In: Richmond R, ed. Educating medical students about tobacco: Planning and implementation. Paris, France: Tobacco Prevention Section, Int. Union Against Tuberculosis and Lung Disease; 1996:61-84

CHAPTER 5b

HELPING RESISTANT SMOKERS QUIT

FOR REFLECTION

How can you deal with a patient who does not respond to quit-smoking advice?

OVERVIEW

Health education and advice approaches prepare you to help 10%-20% of smokers who are ready to quit. Most smoking cessation programs, however, do not adequately address how to deal with resistant, ambivalent, or indifferent smokers. This chapter will help you learn how to motivate such patients to change over time. It discusses how the six-step approach can be used to motivate patients in different stages of the change process, and will provide examples of specific questions you can use with your patients to help them quit smoking

HELPING RESISTANT SMOKERS QUIT

In developing new skills, it helps to start with less severe problems: in this case, smokers who are in the contemplation or preparation stage. After developing some basic skills, you can then begin to work with smokers who are in the precontemplation stage. Although these patients are more challenging to work with, they provide the best opportunities for understanding the change process, even though your chances of short-term success is much less than when dealing with smokers in the contemplation or preparation stage.

STEP 1: BUILDING PARTNERSHIPS

The three component parts of this step are crucial for establishing effective partnerships with patients. This process provides the foundation for helping patients to change.

A. Develop Empathy

Communication Skills for Developing Empathy	
Use open-ended questions	*"How does smoking help you?"*
Use reflective listening	*"So, smoking helps you relax and deal with stressful situations."*
Paraphrase	*"And smoking helps soothe your stress and anger away?"*
Validate feelings	*"I can understand why you would feel angry in those situations."*
Normalize behaviors	*"It's normal to want those angry feelings to go away."*
Affirm strengths	*"It takes courage to keep your angry feelings under control."*
Use probing questions	*"How could you control your angry feelings without smoking?"*

B. Use Relational Skills Effectively

Put the Patient in the One-up Position: *"Tell me what convinces you that you will not become addicted to smoking." "What makes you think that you could give up any time you wanted?" "Is there anything that would convince you to quit now?" "You say you could quit, but what's stopping you from doing it?"*
Take the One-Down Position with a Patient: *"I am not sure a) what it would take to convince you about the real risk of heart disease, b) what more you would like to know about smoking that might convince you to quit, or c) what it would take to convince you about the need to quit."*

C. Clarify Roles and Responsibilities

Clarifying Your Roles
Clarify your prevention role: *"Smoking can damage your health without causing any symptoms. Can I help you protect your health from further damage?"* Clarify the difference between a motivational role (helping patients consider change) and an action-oriented role (treating nicotine addiction): *"I can work with you to help you think more about quitting and increase your chance of setting a quit date (motivational role)."* Or *"Nicotine replacement treatments increase your chance of quitting for good, and I advise you to use one when you set your quit date ('fix-it' role)."*

Clarifying Your Responsibility
"I'll tell you what I know about the risks and harmful effects related to nicotine addiction and smoking, but we may still see the benefits, risks, and harm of smoking differently. If you are willing to work with me on how we see things differently, I may be able to help you increase your motivation to quit. Is that okay?"

STEP 2: NEGOTIATING AN AGENDA

Agenda-setting skills are particularly important because some patients are reluctant or ambivalent about discussing their smoking habit. It is important for you to be sensitive when approaching these patients to avoid evoking undue defensiveness, negative emotions (e.g., anger, irritation), and resistance. The questions and comments in the following tables (prevention- and problem-focused approaches) can help you prevent such reactions from patients.

A. Prevention-focused Approach
This approach is used when patients who do not have any medical problems caused by their tobacco use present with complaints.

Consent-gaining Direct Questions
About smoking: *"I would like to see if there is anything you can do to improve your health. Is it all right to talk about your smoking?"* [Let patient respond.] You can then ask, *"Is there anything that you want to discuss about your smoking, or anything else?"* About quitting: *"I'd like to talk about whether you are interested in quitting. Is that all right?"* [Let patient respond.] You can then ask, *"Is there anything that you want to discuss about your smoking, or anything else?"*
Leading Questions
"Do you want to continue smoking, at least for the time being?" *"Would you consider yourself a die-hard smoker?"* *"Do you think that you will continue smoking for the rest of your life?"*

Prefacing Statements Followed by Challenging Questions
"I would like to talk to you about your smoking in ways that may help you think about it differently. Is that okay?" [Choose any of the following.] *"Tobacco companies are trying to control your behavior by selling you images about smoking. What are those images? Which of them are important to you?* [Let patient respond.] *In what way is that image more important to you than your health?"* *"Tobacco companies benefit if you let yourself become addicted to nicotine. What do you think about what the tobacco industry is trying to do to you?"*
Prefacing Statements Focusing on Lack of Concern about Consequences
"Most young people feel that they can give up smoking any time they want to, and certainly before they damage their health. What do you think?" *"Research shows that most young people think that they can give up smoking, but five years later they have become addicted to nicotine and regret that they ever started smoking. What do you think about this research?"* *"Some people are not concerned about how smoking affects their health. What about you?"* *"Many people believe that the complications from smoking won't happen to them. This is a normal response because people do not like to think that they are deliberately harming themselves. What do you think?"* *"Some people get fed up with people telling them to quit smoking. What has your experience been?"*

B. Problem-focused Approach

Prefacing Statements Followed by Questions
"Smoking can prevent your ulcers (or any other smoking-related problem) from healing." [Pause, let patient respond, and if necessary ask:] *"Did you know that?"* [Let patient respond.] *"I think we need to talk about both your ulcer and your smoking. Is that okay?"* *"Most people have tried to quit smoking and experienced withdrawal symptoms. Have you experienced any withdrawal symptoms?"*
Exploratory Questions
Open-ended, linear questions: *"How has your bronchitis affected your smoking?"* Or, *"How has your smoking affected your bronchitis?"* Closed-ended, linear questions: *"Has your chest infection affected how much you smoke?"* *"Is smoking affecting your chest infection?"* *"Does your smoking make your cough worse?"* *"Has your cough made you feel like cutting down on your smoking?"* Circular questions: *"What concerns do your spouse and children have about how smoking affects your health?"*

STEP 3: ASSESSING RESISTANCE AND MOTIVATION

Consider developing your skills to assess patients' readiness to change and how to use a decision balance, in addition to other options listed. In addition to conducting a motivational assessment, you may also have to address the medical complications caused by tobacco use.

A. Motivational Assessment

Readiness to Change—Direct Questions
"Where are you in terms of your smoking? Let me explain." Select any of the following questions, or use them in any sequence that seems compatible with your impression of your patient. *"Are you interested at all in quitting?"* Or, *"Are you not interested in quitting?"* Or, *"Are you thinking about quitting smoking?"* Or, *"Are you ready to quit anytime soon?"* Depending on the patient's response, you may proceed with: A negative response: *"I hear that you are not interested in giving up smoking at the moment. Would you mind sharing with me why you don't want to quit?"* [Let patient respond. If patient gives nonverbal indications that he or she does mind, then proceed.] *"Would you rather leave it for a later time?"*   An unsure response: *"When will you be ready to think more about a quit date?"*   An affirmative response: *"Are you ready to set a quit date?"*
Readiness to Change—Indirect Questions
Select any one or more of the following: *"Do you have any regrets about starting smoking?"* *"What do you think might convince you to quit?"*   *"Do you think that you will ever stop smoking?"*   *"When might you give up smoking?"*   *"What, if anything, would help you to decide to quit smoking?"*

Use a decision balance with the patient

The decision balance is considered an essential component of the motivational assessment. Depending on patients' readiness to change, you can provide a stage-specific rationale to them about why you are using it. This process can increase patient cooperativeness in completing a decision balance, particularly for those patients in precontemplation.

Specific Rationale and Gaining Consent to Use the Decision Balance
Precontemplation: *"You just told me that you were not interested in quitting. Would you mind if we did a decision balance together? It can help me better understand why you do not want to quit."*   *"You just told me that this is not a good time for you to think about quitting. Would you mind if we did a decision balance together? This may help you think about when it might be a good time to think about quitting."*
Contemplation: *"You told me that you are thinking about quitting. Would you mind if we did a decision balance together? It may help you think more about whether to quit or not."*
Preparation: *"You're thinking about quitting soon. If we did a decision balance together, it could help you set a quit date. Is that okay?"*
Action: *"You are ready to set a date to change. If we did a decision balance together, it could help you prevent a relapse after you quit smoking."*

After providing a rationale for using a decision balance, you can then show the patient what it looks like. You can use a decision balance form or draw one out for the patient.

Sharing the Decision Balance with the Patient
"Let me show you what a decision balance looks like. As we use the decision balance, it can help you better understand your reasons to smoke and your reasons to quit. But first (pointing to the top of the left column), what do you like about smoking cigarettes? I would like to make a note of what you say. Is that okay? You can keep this decision balance to use when you go home if you like."

After gaining the patient's cooperation in doing this task, you can ask one or more questions from each quadrant in the sequence suggested below.

To Quit or Not to Quit: That Is the Question	
1. Benefits of smoking *"What do you like about smoking? And what else?"*	2. Concerns about smoking *"What concerns you about your smoking?"* *"What concerns do others have about your smoking?"*
3. Concerns about quitting *"What concerns do you have if you were to quit?"* *"What effects would quitting have on you?"*	4. Benefits of quitting *"How do you think your health would improve if you were to quit?"* *"In what ways would you benefit from quitting?"*

The primary intent of the assessment is not to help patients decide whether to quit, but to identify benefits and concerns about smoking and quitting without implying they should quit smoking. This approach can give you an insight into the reasons patients smoke in spite of the associated risks and harm.

The table below is an example of a patient's response to a practitioner using the decision balance. These responses can help you individualize how to use motivational interventions with a patient; examples of these interventions are provided in subsequent tables.

Reasons to smoke (Cons)	Reasons to change (Pros)
Benefits of smoking Pleasurable Enjoy smoking after meals Makes me feel relaxed Enjoy smoking when drinking beer	Concerns about smoking Delays healing of ulcer Feel short of breath on exercise Children don't like my smoking Smoking too much makes me feel bad
Concerns about quitting Difficulty in dealing with stress Weight gain Withdrawal symptoms	Benefits of quitting Stops my breathing problem from getting worse Family will be pleased
Resistance	Motivation

Once your patients have completed the decision balance, you can then go on to ask them to provide scores for their motivation and resistance.

Explaining and Obtaining Resistance and Motivation Scores
"The left-hand column represents your reasons to smoke (resistance to change). The right-hand column represents your reasons to change (motivation to quit). On a scale of 0 to 10, 0 meaning none and 10 meaning very high, what score would you give for your reasons to stay the same? [pointing to the left column] *And what score would you give for your reasons to change? Are your resistance and motivation scores based on what you think or feel about change? How would you score your resistance and motivation based on what you feel or think?"*

Use a decision balance with family members

If family members accompany the patient, you can ask them to do a decision balance separately. Afterward, they can compare their perspectives. A family member's decision balance can help you understand how the patient and family members differ in their views about the benefits and concerns of smoking and why they are at different stages of change. When family members are in the action stage (with regard to the patient's smoking habit) and the patient is still in the contemplation stage, family members may nag the patient to change (or be perceived as nagging) and evoke patient resistance toward change.

Negative family influence, such as nagging behavior, is associated with lower smoking cessation rates.[1] The decision balance can help family members understand the patient's resistance and ambivalence about change, but, more important, can help them to stop nagging the patient. Such behavior may cause the patient to regress to the stage of precontemplation; in other words, to stop thinking about quitting or even increase the number of cigarettes smoked per day to relieve this family-caused stress.

At the end of the encounter, you can give the decision balance back to the patient and family members. The patient can then add more to his or her decision balance, perhaps in discussion with another family member, as part of an assignment for the next appointment. This task is intended to help patients think more about their smoking and to clarify their ambivalence about change. This activity can provide additional information that can help you summarize the patient's ambivalence and/or highlight discrepancies between the patient's behavior and some aspect of the patient's self-interest.

Assess motives, competing priorities, energy and self-efficacy

All these factors can influence a patient's motivation level.

Assess Motives
"Tell me what would make you decide to quit, if anything?" [Let patient respond, and with prompting, choose any one or more of the following]: *"Would you quit because family and friends want you to?"*   *"Would you quit because you felt that you ought to change for your health or any other reason?"*   *"Would you quit because it is important to you, or perhaps for a combination of reasons?"*   *"Which is most important?"*
Assess Competing Priorities and Energy
"What competing priorities make it difficult for you to quit?"   *"On a scale of zero to ten, how much energy are you willing to devote to quitting?"*   *"What is distracting you from putting more energy into quitting?"*
Assess Confidence and Ability (self-efficacy)
"On a scale of zero to ten, how would you rate your confidence to quit smoking?"   *"On a scale of zero to ten, how would you rate your ability to quit smoking?"*

Assess supports and barriers

If you can foster support, you can help maintain the patient's motivation.[2] Social influence can also enhance maintenance or reduce the prospects of relapse.[3] Another predictor of relapse following cessation among adults is the smoking habits of friends and family.[4]

Assess Supports
"What kind of help, if any, would help you quit?"   *"Who or what could help you quit?"*   *"Do you know of any community programs you can attend to help you quit?"*

You can also help patients identify external factors (barriers) that contribute to smoking relapse; for example, drinking alcohol, enjoying a cigarette at the end of the meal, participating in leisure activities with friends who smoke,[5] and nagging family members. Sometimes, the absence of negative interactions related to smoking may be more important than the presence of positive social support.[1]

Assess Barriers
"Are there smokers around you who would make it more difficult for you to quit?" *"Do family members and friends nag you about your smoking?"* *"What is hindering you from quitting?"* *"What is making it difficult for you to quit?"*

B. Disease-centered Assessment

The smoking history of the patient is an important, information-gathering component of the disease-focused assessment, in addition to identifying and assessing specific problems caused by smoking.

Smoking History
"How many cigarettes do you smoke a day?" *"How long have you been smoking?"* *"At what age did you start smoking?"* *"Would you be prepared to keep a diary of your smoking to learn more about your habit?"*
Nicotine Addiction and Withdrawal Symptoms
"How soon after getting up do you have your first cigarette?" [Smoking within 30 minutes of waking is indicative of addiction] *"What is the longest period of time during which you were able to stop smoking? Did you experience any withdrawal symptoms?"* *"When you stopped smoking, did it affect you in any way?"* *"Would you be prepared to fill out this questionnaire to assess whether you might benefit from nicotine replacement therapy?"*
Quit Attempts
"How many times have you been able to quit smoking? What did you learn from trying to give up smoking? What caused you to start smoking again?"

STEP 4: ENHANCING MUTUAL UNDERSTANDING

A. Educate Patients about Tobacco Use

Practitioner-centered and patient-centered ways of providing health education about smoking risks and harm are described to highlight how you can deliver information to patients differently. The use of scare tactics to educate patients about the risks and harm of smoking has the potential to be counterproductive by evoking powerful defense mechanisms or resistance behaviors that avoid or minimize health concerns.[6;7] Self-confidence, not fear, has been linked to success in smoking cessation.[8]

Practitioner-centered Education

Traditionally, the practitioner-centered approach involves educating and advising patients about the consequences of smoking, and telling them to quit. These behavior change messages can be delivered in either a threatening or a nonthreatening manner, without really knowing whether the patient already knows the content of the message, or even wants to hear more about it. High-threat communications may elicit statements of agreement from the patients but no change in their behavior. This controlling style of educating patients is a form of practitioner-centered education. When you convey such an informative message in a calm voice, that is autonomy-supportive education.

Practitioner-centered Education
"Most smokers—80%—know many of the harmful effects of smoking, but because they don't know all the harmful effects, they tend to underestimate the hazards of smoking.[9] *Most people know that smoking causes lung cancer, but they may not know that smoking kills more patients through heart disease than does all cancers, including lung cancer, and that it is responsible for 89% of chronic bronchitis and emphysema.*"[10;11]
Risks of smoking: *"Smoking is damaging your lungs without causing you any symptoms. It takes many years before you develop symptoms of lung disease."* [Let patient respond.]
Harmful effects of smoking: *"Not only has smoking caused your breathing problem, but it will eventually make it much worse. It is just a question of time before you won't be able to walk one hundred yards before having to catch your breath."* [Let patient respond.]
Provide educational booklets if patient would like them: *"Here are some pamphlets about quitting and using nicotine replacement treatments."*
Educate patients about nicotine withdrawal symptoms: *"When you stop smoking, it may cause a number of symptoms during the first couple of weeks.* [use all or select any of the following as examples]: *anxiety, inadequate sleep, irritability, impatience, difficulty concentrating, restlessness, craving for tobacco, hunger, gastrointestinal problems, headaches, and/or drowsiness."*
Educate patients about nicotine replacement therapy: *"Nicotine treatment, such as gum, the patch, or a nasal inhaler, reduces the withdrawal symptoms and the urge to smoke. This treatment prevents relapses, particularly during the first few weeks after quitting, but it alone will not cure you of your smoking habit. You will still crave cigarettes after you stop using this treatment. Successful quitting still depends on your willpower. Would you like more information about using this treatment to help you over the first four to eight weeks?"*

Patient-centered Education

Health education using the same messages described above also becomes more patient-centered if you ask patients if they would like more information and/or pamphlets, tailor your messages to meet their needs, or deliver such messages in a personally meaningful way.

Patient-centered Education about Risk and Harm
Risks of smoking: *"At the moment you are not noticing any problems caused by your smoking, but are you aware of the health problems caused by smoking?"* [Let patient respond, and then provide additional information that you think patient is most interested in hearing.] *"Unfortunately, smoking damages people's lungs long before they develop lung cancer, and also puts them at an increased risk of developing heart disease, but again, without causing any symptoms. If you are concerned about any breathing problems, would you like me to do some simple tests (peak flow meter) to check up on this?"* [Let patient respond. With a negative answer, ask the patient why he or she is not interested in this suggestion; with a positive answer, proceed.]   Harmful effects of smoking: *"I'm concerned that your smoking has not only caused your breathing problem, but that it's making it much worse, as you know. What concerns do you have about how your shortness of breath will interfere with what it is important for you to do?"* [Let patient respond.]

Alternatively, you can initially focus on the beneficial aspects of smoking and then provide information that helps patients see the benefits less favorably. For example, smoking cigarettes has beneficial effects (pleasure, relaxation, and stress reduction) that are not entirely due to the drug effects of nicotine.

Patient-centered Education about Nicotine
Educating patients about nicotine addiction: *"You said that you find smoking pleasurable. However, it is quite complicated to understand how nicotine affects you. Nicotine is a stimulant. When you first smoke a cigarette, it gives you a sense of alertness and also increases your heart rate. After this effect wears off, you get a relaxed feeling. But it is important for you to realize that this relaxed feeling is not all due to nicotine. The tobacco companies advertise cigarette smoking as a relaxing activity. In fact, your belief that smoking is relaxing may be just as important as the effect of nicotine. In other words, you have a greater ability to relax than you realize, but the advertisers deceive you into thinking that it is all due to nicotine."*   Smoking cigarettes deceives patients about its beneficial effects (relaxation and stress reduction): *"If you're physically addicted to nicotine, you will experience mild withdrawal symptoms, such as feeling stressed or tense, a few hours after not having a cigarette. Cigarette smoking is incredibly deceptive because it makes you think that smoking helps you feel relaxed and relieves your stress, but you're just treating your withdrawal symptoms without knowing it. Does this make sense to you?"* [For patients who need further explanation] *"Let me see if I can explain it another way. Smoking cigarettes is like a vicious circle. Nicotine makes you first feel alert but as this effect wears off, you feel relaxed. After a while, you get withdrawal symptoms and start to feel tense or stressed. So, you smoke a cigarette to relieve those*

Patient-centered Education about Nicotine
feelings. It can be difficult to know whether those tense feelings are due to the withdrawal symptoms or due to the stresses you are under. Nicotine teaches you that you need to smoke to cope with tension and stress, but these feelings may just be due to nicotine withdrawal." Nicotine addiction convinces some patients to believe that they have no willpower to quit: *"You say that you have no willpower to quit, but you may not understand your nicotine addiction. Nicotine addiction may be stronger than your willpower to quit, but that doesn't mean that you have no willpower. There are a number of ways to treat nicotine addiction—the gum and patch are available over the counter from drugstores. These treatments help you overcome your withdrawal syndrome, but the real test is whether you are willing to use these treatments and put your willpower to the test. I can also work with you to help you build up your willpower to quit for life, but it may take many attempts to do it. People who succeed don't quit trying to quit."*

B. Use Nondirect Interventions to Lower Resistance

You can use nondirect interventions to understand why patients do not want to quit and to help patients lower their resistance to quitting.

Nondirect Interventions to Lower Resistance
Use simple reflection to elicit ambivalence: *"So, you are getting more short of breath when exercising."* Or, *"So, your family is concerned about the effects of smoking on your breathing."*
Probe priorities to explore ambivalence: *"So, what do you like most about smoking? And what concerns you most about your smoking?"*   *"What concerns you most about quitting? What do you think would be the most important benefit of quitting?"*
Use double-sided reflection to summarize ambivalence: *"On the one hand, you said that smoking helps you relax, but on the other hand, it is making you feel short of breath when you go for walks."*
Acknowledge ambivalence: *"You seem to have mixed feelings about your smoking; you smoke to relax, but your kids are concerned about your smoking."*
Emphasize personal responsibility and choice (useful when patients are being resistant): *"What you decide to do about smoking is entirely up to you, but I'll help you if you would like."*
Explore the future: *"So, what was your breathing like five years ago when you were smoking, compared to now? What do you think your breathing will be like in five years?"*

C. Use Direct Interventions to Motivate Change

Direct interventions help patients confront themselves, such that they change their perceptions and values about their smoking and their health. This process helps patients enhance their motivation to change.

Back-to-the-Future Questions
"How short of breath would you have to get before you would decide to quit smoking?" [Provided that patient shows some interest in prevention, continue.] *"Do you want to wait and see if this happens before you decide to quit?"* [If patient remains interested in prevention, continue:] *"What would really convince you to quit?"* [If patient is ambivalent, or not interested in prevention, ask:] *"Would you mind sharing with me why you don't want to quit?"*

Benefit Substitution
"What other ways do you use to help you relax, other than smoking?" *"Can you reward yourself in other ways rather than smoking a cigarette?"*

Clarifying Values
Questions that probe values: *"So, what is more important in your life than smoking (or your health)?"* Questions that contrast values: *"Smoking to relax is more important to you than your lungs and avoiding breathing problems."* *"The pleasure of smoking is worth more than the risk to your health."* Questions that contrast values and behavior: *"If you say that your lungs are more important than smoking to relax, you're saying one thing and doing another. What would convince you to do what you say?"*

Challenging Rationalizations
"Do you mind if I say a few things that might help you think about your smoking differently?" [With an affirmative response from the patient] *"It may make you pause and even feel a little uncomfortable, but I am just trying to help you think about whether you would like to improve your health. You don't have to say anything if you don't feel like it, and if you want me to quit talking about it, just tell me."* [Choose any of the following approaches.]
"Most young people don't think that they will become addicted to nicotine, but five years later, most of them regret that they ever started smoking. What do you think?" *"Many people believe that they won't die from smoking complications, and that protects them from really thinking about how they are damaging their own health."* [Be silent; if necessary, prompt with a follow-up comment or question.]
"Many people say that they have to die some time from something, but that depends on whether they have more important things to live for, other than smoking." [Be silent; if necessary, prompt with a follow-up comment or question.] *"You say that you don't care if you die, but are you concerned about the quality of your life before you die?"*

"Smoking helps you deal with your stress, but you're dealing with that stress much better than you think you are. Nicotine first acts as a stimulant, but, as it wears off, it makes you feel relaxed and able to cope with stress better. What may be more important than this effect is your belief that smoking helps relieve your stress. Your mind may be more powerful than nicotine to help you cope with stress. When smokers stop and have a cigarette, they do a number of other things at the same time to cope with stress. They may take a timeout, sit down, and maybe say to themselves: 'I deserve a cigarette to relax.' Everything you do at the same time as having a cigarette may be more powerful in relieving your stress than nicotine. What do you think about that?" [Pause, and let the patient respond.] *You're doing a much better job of coping with your stress than you think you are. The problem is that you're kidding yourself that only smoking is helping you relax (or cope with stress). What would it take for you to relax (or deal with this stress), but without kidding yourself that smoking is doing it?"*

Discrepancies
Identify discrepancies: *"You say that smoking helps you relax."* [Let patient acknowledge your comments nonverbally.] *"But it makes your family worry about your health."* [Let patient respond. Help patient develop his or her own discrepancies: *"You say that you exercise and smoke to relax. Do you see any inconsistency with how you are trying to relax?"*
Reframing Items, Issues or Events
Change a reason to smoke into a reason not to smoke: *"You enjoy smoking, but how does your cough feel in the morning?"* Enhance a reason to quit smoking: *"Your kids are concerned about your smoking. If you quit, they won't worry about your health. What's more, you will be in a better position to help your kids when they become teenagers and are at risk of developing a smoking habit."* Diminish a reason to smoke: *"You enjoy smoking after meals, but that delays the healing of your ulcer."*
Challenging Claims or Positions
Use amplified reflection: *"So, you are not worried at all about the complications of smoking or dying? And you are not worried at all about how smoking affects the quality of your life before you die?" "So, you are not concerned at all that your children are worried about your smoking and health?"*
Differences in Motivational Reasons
"You take your tablets on a regular basis to control your hypertension [integrated motivation]. *You feel that you ought to lose weight* [introjected motivation] *but you only exercise when your wife goes with you* [extrinsic motivation]. *Nor do you seem interested in quitting* [indifferent motivation]. *What would it take for you to lose weight, exercise, and quit smoking in the same way that you take care of yourself by taking your tablets regularly?"* [Let the patient respond.] *"In fact, you would do your health more good by quitting cigarettes than by taking your tablets regularly."*

Monitoring Changes in Resistance and Motivation Scores
"What scores would you now give for your resistance and motivation, using the scale of 0-10? "Why did you change your resistance score? And why did you change your motivation score?" "You can learn a lot about yourself even if your scores got worse and went in the wrong

Monitoring Changes in Resistance and Motivation Scores
direction. Sometimes it helps if your resistance score goes up and your motivation score goes down as it can teach you what it would take to change for good."

D. Clarify Differences in Perception about Patient Self-efficacy

Once you have reached this stage in assessing patient motivation, it is a good idea to assess your and your patient's perception of this motivation before moving on to implement a plan for change. This enables both you and your patient to be at the same stage of change.

Asking about Confidence and Ability (Self-efficacy)
"We've been working together, and I would like you to think about your score on a scale of zero to ten. How would you now rate your ability (and/or confidence) to quit smoking?" [Let patient respond.] Address whether you agree with your patient's self-assessment or not.

Clarifying Persistent Differences in Perceptions
"I think it is important for us to be clear about how we see the benefits, risks and harm of smoking—the same or differently—because that will affect how we work together. I think I understand what you like about smoking, but I seem more concerned about the risks and harms caused by your smoking than you are. What do you think?"

STEP 5: IMPLEMENTING A PLAN FOR CHANGE

This step requires working with your patients toward a plan for change, establishing realistic goals, and working toward their implementation.

A. Evaluate Patient Commitment toward a Plan of Change

A number of factors can influence a patient's commitment to the change process.

Evaluating Commitment from the Perspective of Competing Priorities
"What is going on in your life that makes it difficult for you to quit now? Anything else? What would it take for you to put 'quit smoking' at the top of your list of things to do?"
Evaluating Commitment from the Perspective of Patient's Energy
"What is going on that makes it difficult for you to devote your energy to quitting?"   *"What would it take for you to put your energy into quitting?"*   *"If you don't have any energy to quit, what would it take for you to get your energy back?"*
Evaluating Commitment from the Perspective of Motivational Reasons
"What makes you commit yourself to quit. And what else?" "You say that you are here because your girlfriend wanted you to come. What would it take for you to come for your own reasons?"

B. Decide on Goals

The table below lists a range of goals for change that you can give your patients.

Range of Goals
• Think more about quitting. Use a decision balance to consider quitting.
• Prepare for change. Plan how to quit, learn about nicotine addiction and withdrawal, inform family and friends about plans to quit, and use the decision balance to build willpower to change.
• Set a quit date.
• Additional options: Nicotine replacement therapy, referral to smoking cessation programs, referral to a counselor for associated problems such as relational conflicts.

Practitioners can selectively use nicotine replacement therapy to treat patients' withdrawal syndromes and thereby increase the smoking cessation rates. While nicotine replacement therapy is invaluable for treating patients' short-term physical addiction (1 to 2 weeks), however, the one-year recidivism rate is high without the concurrent use of behavioral methods.[12-16]

Goal-setting

You can set up goals for change in one of three ways:

1. Practitioner-selected goals

In this scenario, the practitioner takes control of goal-setting, using one of the two following approaches:

An authoritarian, advice-giving monologue: *"You should quit smoking now before you further damage your lungs."*

An authoritative, advice-giving monologue: *"Smoking is damaging your lungs and making you more short of breath when you run. I recommend that you quit smoking, but that's up to you."*

2. Patient-selected goals

Most patients quit smoking without seeking professional help. They decide whether or not they are going to think about quitting, and how long they are willing to stay in the different stages of change. You can act as a catalyst, however, to accelerate the pace of change.

An engaging monologue: *"You seemed concerned when we talked about your father developing emphysema that was made worse by his smoking. You are now concerned that you are repeating family history because you are getting more short of breath when you run. But you can change the course of family history if you choose to learn from your father. He was told too late to quit smoking because the tobacco companies did not put warning labels on cigarette packages. What do you want to do about your smoking? Prefer not to think about it? Think about it some more? Prepare yourself to quit, or set a quit date?"*

3. Negotiated approach to goal setting

An engaging dialogue:

MP: *"I am concerned because your father developed emphysema, and he quit smoking only one year before he died. And now, you're getting short of breath when you run. What do you think about your family history?"*

Patient: *"Well, my grandfather never gave up smoking and he died from lung disease."*

MP, half-jokingly: *"I suppose you have thought about whether it was worth it for your father to quit smoking since he died a year later. He could have enjoyed smoking for another year."*

Patient: *"That was what my brother said to my dad a week before he died. My dad had one cigarette just before he died. He inhaled it only once. He was too exhausted to smoke it."*

MP: *"Even though it did not benefit your father, perhaps he gave you a gift by quitting to help future generations. What can you learn from your father about changing family history?"*

Patient: *"I need to quit, but I am not ready to now. I have not recovered from my dad's death."*

MP in a low-key tone of voice: *"So, smoking will help you recover from this stress?"*

Patient: *"Yes...no, not really."*

MP: *"Are you willing to think more about quitting, or even to prepare for a quit date?"*

Patient: *"I think that I will try to quit in six weeks, on my fiftieth birthday."*

C. Work toward Solutions[17]

You can use the MED-STAT acronym to help your patients implement a plan.

Interventions	Solution-based Approaches to Implementing a Plan
Miracle question (explore change)	*"Suppose a miracle happened and you quit smoking tomorrow. What would your life be like? How would your family and friends respond?"*
Exceptions (identify strengths)	*"What goes on when you smoke less compared to times when you smoke more than usual?"* Or, *"What's going on when you are stressed, but you don't smoke a cigarette?"*
Difference (use strengths)	*"What makes a difference when you smoke less rather than more? How can you apply your experiences when you don't smoke and you are stressed to those situations when you do smoke when you are stressed?"*
Scaling (assess motivation, self-efficacy and outcome expectancy)	*"On a scale of zero to ten, how would you rate your (motivation, competence, or confidence) to quit? How would you rate whether you can achieve your goal for change (outcome expectancy)? What would increase or decrease your scores? Can you make a list of those things? Was there a time when your scores were higher than now? What would it take to tip the balance in favor of higher scores?"*
Timeouts (consider alternatives)	*"What ideas do you have about how you could handle your stress differently other than smoking?"* Check out silences. *"A moment ago, I asked you a question and you were silent. What was going on?"*
Accolades (enhance efficacy)	*"You clearly have the skills to quit, but what would it take for you to keep using your skills?"*
Task appraisals (encourage action)	*"What would it take for you to think more about quitting, or to quit smoking sooner rather than later? When would be a good time to quit?"*

STEP 6: FOLLOWING THROUGH

Once the patient has decided to think about quitting, or to actually quit, it is important to continue to motivate him or her by following up on a plan of action in order to prevent lapses or a relapse.

A. Rationale, Purpose and Reasons for Follow-up
You can encourage the patient to make follow-up appointments, to keep track of change.

Providing Rationale for Follow-up
"I think it's important for you to come back and discuss [choose one or more of the following]: *how your smoking is affecting your health; how to overcome nicotine addiction; or, how to deal with the complications from your smoking."* [And then decide whether to set up a follow-up appointment.]
Clarifying Patients' Reasons to Attend Follow-up
"Why is it important for you to attend a follow-up appointment? What do you think is the most important reason for you to attend a follow-up appointment? What health concerns do you want to address at your next appointment?"

B. Arrange Follow-up

Arranging Follow-up
"Would you like to come back for a follow-up appointment?"
"How soon do you want to come back and check up on your health concern?"
"I think it's important for you to decide when to come back for a follow-up appointment. I will certainly share what I think about this, but I'm more interested in what you think."

C. Use Methods to Ensure Change
Behavior modification may involve one of two divergent approaches: negative and positive reinforcement.[18] An aversive approach that is relatively effective involves the patient increasing the number of cigarettes smoked and the rate at which they are smoked.[19] Positive reinforcement that includes self-management procedures (monitoring urges, developing strategies for dealing with temptations, and contracting) has limited success.[1;20-25] You can use a diary, relapse prevention strategies, and motivational reevaluation approaches to ensure that patients maintain change.

1. A diary to track thoughts, feelings and behavior over time

A Diary for Tracking Change
"Are you interested in keeping a diary to understand your smoking habit better so that you can anticipate when you are likely to relapse after quitting? It would also help if you were to record your thoughts and feelings during situations when you feel tempted to smoke."

2. Relapse prevention approach

One limitation of the relapse prevention approach is that patients who maintain cessation compared with those who relapse have similar skills for coping with stresses; people who relapse, however, do not use their coping skills at times of heightened vulnerability.[3] In essence, patients relapse not because of a lack of skills but from a failure to use their skills. Consequently, approaches to help patients develop relapse prevention skills may be unwarranted if patients lack sustained motivation to use the skills they have. Studies that have examined relapse prevention strategies are, at best, only moderately encouraging.[1:26] Some strategies are listed below.

Relapse Prevention Approach
Management of risk situations: *"The physical urges to smoke are worse during the first two weeks of the withdrawal syndrome, but the psychological cravings for cigarettes can persist for months or years after smoking. In what situations are you likely to start smoking again? How about making a list of how to deal with those urges and cravings?"*   Pharmacological management: *"How do you think you will benefit from nicotine replacement therapy? Do you have any concerns about using nicotine replacement therapy?"*   Emotional management: *"When you feel stressed (or any other negative emotions), how do you think you can deal with those feelings other than by lighting up a cigarette?"*   Reevaluation of supports: *"Would it help to have someone help you quit?"*   Reevaluation of barriers: *"What do you think is making it difficult for you to quit? How do you think you're going to handle those difficulties?"*   Use of positive reinforcement: *"Would it be helpful you to set up a reward for quitting? What would that be?"*

C. Motivational Reevaluation

When patients have lapsed, relapsed or are struggling to maintain change, you can revisit their decision balance to reassess their "think" and "feeling" scores for their resistance and motivation.

Motivational Reevaluation
"Let's look again at your decision balance so you can tell me how your 'think' and 'feeling' scores for your resistance and motivation are changing. [Let patient respond] What's making your resistance score go up and your motivation score go down? [Let patient respond] What could help to make your scores better?"

MOVING ON

This chapter described a motivational approach to smoking cessation that you can use when quit smoking advice does not work. Chapter 6a addresses the issue of multiple agendas involved in the self-care of diabetes.

Reference List

1. Antonuccio DO, Boutilier LR, Ward CH, et al. The behavioral treatment of cigarette smoking. Progress in Behavior Modification 1992;28: 119-181

2. Fisher EB, Jr., Haire-Joshu D, Morgan GD, et al. Smoking and smoking cessation. American Review of Respiratory Disease 1990;142: 702-720

3. Fisher EB, Jr., Rost K. Smoking cessation: a practical guide for the physician. Clinics in Chest Medicine 1986;7: 551-565

4. Fisher EB, Jr., Fondren DP. Undirected smoking cessation: A survey of successful quitters. Washington University; 1986

5. Shiffman S. A cluster-analytic classification of smoking relapse episodes. Addictive Behaviors 1986;11: 295-307

6. Job RFS. Effective and ineffective use of fear in health promotion campaigns. American Journal of Public Health 1988;78: 163-167

7. Orleans CT. Understanding and promoting smoking cessation: Overview and guidelines for physician intervention. Annual Review of Medicine 1985;36: 51-61

8. Condiotte MM, Lichtenstein E. Self-efficacy and relapse in smoking cessation programs. Journal of Consulting and Clinical Psychology 1981;49: 648-658

9. U.S.Department of Health & Human Services. Reducing the Health Consequences of Smoking: 25 Years of Progress: A Report of the Surgeon General (DHHS publication No. [CDC] 89-8411). Rockville, MD: U.S. Government Printing Office; 1989

10. U.S.Department of Health & Human Services. The health consequences of smoking: Chronic obstructive lung disease: A report of the Surgeon General (DHHS publication No. [PHS] 84-50205). Rockville, MD: U.S. Government Printing Office; 1984

11. U.S.Department of Health & Human Services. The health consequences of smoking: Cardiovascular disease: A report of the Surgeon General (DHHS Publication No. [PHS] 84-50204). Washington, DC: Office on Smoking and Health; 1984

12. Tonnesen P, Norregaard J, Simonsen K, et al. A double-blind trial of a 16-hour transdermal nicotine patch in smoking cessation. New England Journal of Medicine 1991;325: 311-315

13. Wong JG. How to help your patients quit smoking: Strategies that work. Postgraduate Medicine 1993;94: 197-201

14. Miller GH, Golish JA, Cox CE. A physician's guide to smoking cessation. Journal of Family Practice 1992;34: 759-760, 762-766

15. Benowitz NL, Jacob P, Savanapridi C. Determinants of nicotine intake while chewing nicotine polacrilex gum. Clinical Pharmacology & Therapeutics 1987;41: 467-473

16. Blum A. Nicotine chewing gum and the medicalization of smoking. Annals of Internal Medicine 1984;101: 121-123

17. Giorlando ME, Schilling RJ. On becoming a solution-focused physician: The MED-STAT acronym. Families, Systems & Health 1997;15: 361-373

18. Schwartz JL. Methods of smoking cessation. Med Clin North Am 1992;76: 451-476

19. Danaher BG. Research on rapid smoking: Interim summary and recommendations. Addictive Behaviors 1977;2: -151

20. Glasgow RE. Smoking. In: Holroyd K, Creer T, eds. Self-management of chronic disease and handbook of clinical interventions and research. Orlando, FL: Academic Press; 1986:99

21. Lichtenstein E, Brown RA. Current trends in the modification of cigarette dependence. In: Bellak AS, Hersen M, Kazdin AE, eds. International Handbook of Behavior Modification and Therapy. New York, NY: Plenum Press; 1983:575

22. Pechacek TF. Modification of smoking behavior. In: Krasnegor NA, ed. The behavioral aspects of smoking (NIDA Res Monogr 26) (DHEW publication No. 79-882). Bethesda: U.S. Department of Health, Education and Welfare; 1979:127

23. Schwartz JL. Smoking cures: Ways to kick an unhealthy habit. In: Jarvik ME, Cullen JW, Gritz ER, et al., eds. Research in smoking behavior (NIDA Research Monogr 17) (DHEW publication No. [ADM] 78-581). Bethesda: U.S. Department of Health, Education and Welfare; 1977:308-335

24. Schwartz JL. Review and evaluation of smoking cessation methods: The United States and Canada. [DHHS publication no. 87-2940]. Rockville, MD: National Cancer Institute, Department of Health and Human Services; 1987

25. Schwartz JL, Dubitzky M. Requisites for success in smoking withdrawal. In: Borgatta EF, Evans RR, eds. Smoking, health, & behavior. Chicago, IL: Aldine Publishing; 1968:231-247

26. Curry SJ, McBride CM. Relapse prevention for smoking cessation: review and evaluation of concepts and interventions. Annu Rev Public Health 1994;15: 345-366

CHAPTER 6a

DIABETES

FOR REFLECTION

How can you help patients address the multiple tasks of caring for diabetes?
What factors help patients to adhere to the goals of self-care?

OVERVIEW

This chapter provides some key facts as well as a primer on specific issues that promote or hinder self-care of diabetes. This self-care involves adherence to multiple tasks to prevent complications for patients or to reduce the impact of these complications on them. These tasks vary according to what phase of diabetes the patient is in.

Early Phase

Work toward normal blood glucose levels and Hb A1c—monitor blood glucose regularly; adhere to insulin or drug regimen; adhere to diabetic diet; keep blood pressure below 130/85; reduce weight (if relevant); exercise regularly; monitor cholesterol levels; and stop smoking (if applicable).

Intermediate Phase

Prevent specific complications—schedule appointments for eye exams to detect and treat diabetic retinopathy; inspect feet for neuropathy and vascular insufficiency; adhere to treatment for lowering cholesterol; treat any concomitant cardiovascular risk factors; and treat microalbuminuria with angiotensin-converting enzymes.

Late Phase

Minimize the impact of diabetic complications—use adaptive devices; schedule regular follow-up appointments with specialists; adapt environment to functional decline; understand and adjust to diabetic complications; deal with functional decline; and deal with death and dying issues (living wills, health care proxies).

DIABETES

KEY FINDINGS

Diabetic self-care is important for the following reasons:

- Research shows that improved glycemic control reduces complication rates in Type 1 diabetes.[1-4] The Diabetes Control and Complications Trial (DCCT) study clearly demonstrated that intensive insulin therapy to achieve normoglycemia reduced complication rates. [1;2;5] An approximate 40% risk reduction occurred for each 10% decrease in Hb A1c. However, a 1% decrease at a higher level (from 12% to 11%) decreased absolute risk more than at a lower level (from 8% to 7%).[3] Patients do benefit by reducing their Hb A1c to whatever level they can achieve.

- A Japanese study found that Type II diabetic patients treated with multiple insulin injections, compared to the usual insulin injections, decreased cumulative incidence of retinopathy, nephropathy, and neuropathy in a way that was similar to the DCCT study. A glycemic threshold for fasting blood glucose of 110 mg/dL (6.11 mmol/L) and a 2-hour postprandial blood glucose level of 180 mg/dL (10.0) mmol/L corresponded to an Hb A1c level of 6.5%, below which these complications did not progress. Questions remain about the advantages and disadvantages of intensive insulin therapy of Type II diabetes.[6]

- The recent United Kingdom Prospective Diabetes (Type II) Study (UKPDS) found that more intensive blood pressure control reduced diabetes mortality (number needed to treat = 15 for 10 years to prevent one diabetes-related death) but not overall mortality.[7-12] Major cardiovascular events in Type II diabetes were reduced by blood pressure control with low-dose diuretics, Atenolol, and angiotensin enzyme inhibitors (NNT = 10 to 20 for five to 10 years for primary prevention of one cardiovascular event). Better glycemic control was not related to overall or diabetes-specific mortality, except for obese patients treated with metformin (NNT = 14 for 10 years to prevent one death, and NNT = 19 for 10 years to prevent one diabetes-related death). [13] Control of hypertension reduced microvascular and macrovascular complications more than glycemic control. This conclusion warrants some caution as the mean Hb A1c levels in the control and study groups were 7.7 and 7.0, respectively. The control group had an Hb A1c level that was only 0.7 higher than the study group, suggesting that patients in the control group also had their diabetes in good control.

- DCCT-defined intensive therapy is well within the range of cost effectiveness and considered to represent good value (incremental cost of life gain is $28,661).[14]

- Annual health care costs are 3.6 times higher for diabetic patients. Diabetes accounts for one in seven dollars spent on health care in the United States. The direct cost for confirmed cases is $85 billion, and the total estimated cost is $92-$105 billion.[15]

Additional information about diabetes for practitioners and patients is on Web sites listed at the end of this chapter.

SPECIFIC ISSUES

The efficacy-effectiveness gap is wide in terms of the differences between a health care team conducting research studies in ideal settings and practitioners dealing with patients in real-world practice. Primary care practitioners do not have adequate personnel and infrastructure support to organize disease management programs. Teamwork and quality improvement methods can help health care settings to reduce the efficacy-effectiveness gap and to develop disease management programs in their health care settings.[16] Specialists and generalists also need training in how to motivate patients to take better control of themselves if they are to promote patient adherence to minimize the development of complications.[17;17-21]

A. Relationship of Adherence to Outcomes

Adherence to diabetic recommendations, improved glycemic control, reduced glycosylated hemoglobin, and improved health care outcomes (such as preventable morbidity and mortality, and quality of life) are interrelated in interesting ways (see Figure 6.1, page 150). Glycemic control is an intermediate outcome that reduces the risk of certain complications. Patient adherence to self-care of diabetes guidelines, however, enhances the prospects of, but does not necessarily ensure, normoglycemic control.

Some patients have difficulties in controlling their blood glucose levels even when they adhere to the guidelines. Conversely, normoglycemic control (a normal Hb A1c level) does not necessarily mean that patients fully adhere to the guidelines. For example, patients with Type II diabetes can achieve a normal Hb A1c by weight reduction alone, without exercising or following a diabetic diet.

Diabetic control and adherence may relate positively or negatively to different health care outcomes. Achieving normoglycemic control may encourage patients to adhere to a regimen, particularly if adherence avoids diabetic complications. Some patients, however, do not feel that it is worth the effort to achieve normoglycemic control because of its negative impact on their enjoyment of life (e.g., social consequences, dietary sacrifices). They treasure this enjoyment and minimize concerns about dying from diabetes. Other patients put tremendous effort into diabetic adherence without achieving normoglycemia and without feeling that their quality of life has improved. Not surprisingly, they may become demoralized and stop adhering to the recommendations.

Figure 6.1: Interrelationships of Adherence, Normoglycemia and Outcomes

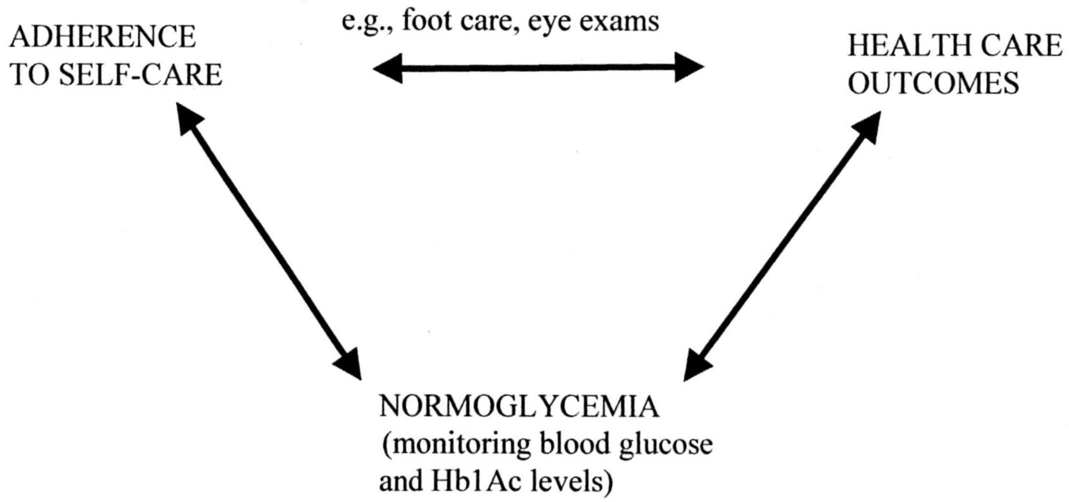

Self-care of diabetes is a challenging, chronic disease because patients have to address multiple tasks to prevent diabetic complications.[22;23] Consequently, patients and practitioners achieve relatively low levels of adherence to the recommended guidelines.[18;24-26] Yet even though patients do more than 90% of diabetic care,[27] your role is significant in helping promote patient adherence. To fulfill this role, you need to be aware of the various factors that may help or hinder a patient's adherence to self-care of diabetes.

B. Factors Affecting Adherence

Adherence to a diabetic regimen involves multiple self-care tasks.[17;19] Research shows that adherence to any one task is not correlated highly to other tasks.[28-31] Thus, patients adhere to their regimen to varying degrees;[31] better to a medical regimen (taking drugs and injecting insulin), for example, than to lifestyle changes, such as diet and exercise.[28;31-34]

Demographic variables

Adherence to diabetic guidelines is not associated with demographic variables such as household income, gender, ethnic group, years of education, marital status, number and length of medical consultations, or patient reports of treatment satisfaction.[35;36] Affluent and low-income patients have similar levels of nonadherence.

This data dispels the idea that you can predict adherence based on demographic characteristics.

Information-giving

Practitioner-patient interactions do affect diabetic adherence.[37] Patients often forget recommendations, particularly if delivered in a vague, complex, or threatening manner.[38;39] Written materials as well as family member involvement in the clinical encounter can help patients remember what they can do to enhance the prospects of avoiding diabetic complications. It is up to you to tailor your communications in ways that help patients to retain information.

Patient knowledge

Educating patients may increase their knowledge about ideal recommendations for self-care of diabetes, but this does *not* necessarily ensure that patients will adhere to them. Furthermore, attempts to help patients improve their self-care have been criticized for relying excessively on the mere provision of information.[40] Interestingly, general knowledge about diabetes is not consistently related to adherence. Some studies even report that knowledge is inversely related to adherence.[37;41;42] It is important to distinguish, however, between abstract medical knowledge and the kinds of information that patients find particularly helpful in trying to solve problems related to self-care of their diabetes.

Developing individualized self-care plans

You can empower patients to take a greater role in caring for their diabetes and to enhance their problem-solving skills.[43;44] After considering the patient's situation, values, needs, readiness to change, preferences, and abilities,[24;45] you can negotiate with patients about goals for change. You can use behavioral interventions (described in Chapter 6b) to help patients achieve their goals. Patients often need assistance from other members of the health care team to work on their goals.[45]

You can help patients work toward the ideal recommendations by developing an individualized self-care regimen. Such an approach is less likely to leave patients feeling overwhelmed and confused. Follow-up support between office visits that provides individualized interventions to patients may also help them work toward and achieve their goals.[46-48] These goals fall into two categories: lifestyle changes and disease monitoring.

C. Need for Lifestyle Changes

There are various options you can encourage patients to choose that will help them to take charge of caring for their diabetes.

Diet

Helping patients adhere to a standard, diabetic diet over the long term is one of the most challenging aspects of promoting self-care of diabetes; patients concur by reporting that diet and exercise are the most difficult aspects of diabetic management.[28] Three-quarters of diabetic patients report deviating significantly from dietary recommendations at least weekly.[40;49] It is important to note that patients may view tasks and the reasons for adherence differently from their practitioners.[34] Such unresolved differences in perspective often perpetuate nonadherence.[50;51] To enhance the prospects of patients adhering to dietary recommendations, the American Diabetes Association has developed a more flexible approach to diets that involves individualized assessment, negotiated goal-setting, problem-solving, and ongoing evaluation.[24;52]

Weight loss

For Type II diabetes, sustained weight loss of at least 15 pounds is needed to improve glycemic control. Even when patients maintain weight loss over time, they may experience deterioration in their glycemic control.[53] Obese, Type 2 diabetic patients also lose less weight and reduce their food intake less than their obese, nondiabetic spouses,[54] and they find it difficult to sustain weight loss over time. Structured and intensive behavioral programs using very low-calorie diets under supervision may help to produce long-term weight loss.[55] The most successful approach to long-term weight control involves programs that combine diet, exercise, and behavior modification.[55-57]

Exercise

Moderate regular exercise is beneficial for both healthy individuals and for patients with chronic disease.[58] Exercise is an adjunct to diet in controlling diabetes.[59] Regular, rigorous exercise helps to increase insulin sensitivity.

D. Monitoring Diabetes

In addition to making lifestyle changes, patients need to actively monitor different aspects of their disease.

Glucose levels and glycosolated hemoglobin

A study of insulin-dependent diabetic children clustered the various aspects of self-care into five domains:

- Insulin injection
- Frequency of eating and glucose monitoring
- Diet type
- Diet amount
- Exercise[30]

To compound the challenge of providing diabetic care, patients (particularly adolescents) often inflate their reports about the number of glucose tests they have done by as much as 50%.[60-63] Such behavior may represent attempts to please their practitioner. Conversely, patients may test themselves less often when the result of the glucose levels does not change in their diabetic regimen.

If you recommend an increase in glucose testing, it is of negligible benefit unless you use the results to change the regimen (e.g., insulin dose and frequency, eating habits, and exercise).[33] Overall, the best measure for assessing glucose control is glycosolated hemoglobin. Patients can have their levels checked every 6-12 weeks depending on their treatment goals.

Unnecessary hospitalizations

Avoiding hospitalization is one goal of self-care of diabetes. For example, failure to administer insulin is a common cause for admission because of diabetic ketoacidosis. More than one-half of patients reported psychological stress as the reason for neglecting their insulin regimen. Social support may help some patients buffer psychological stress in ways that avoid hospitalization.[64]

Complications

Patients and practitioners need to pay attention to the risk of kidney, eye, and foot complications.

- Kidney protection:[65;66] Practitioners may not survey their patients regularly enough to detect microalbuminuria early on. Once it is identified, however, angiotensin-converting enzyme drugs may stop or slow its development.[67;68] Compared to its absence, the presence of microalbuminuria represents a 9-20 times greater risk of developing progressive nephropathy,[69-71] a 15-fold greater risk of dying from cardiovascular disease, and a 148% increased risk of dying from all causes.[72-75] In an 11-year follow-up study, nearly 70% of patients with microalbuminuria developed retinopathy as compared to zero percentage of patients without microalbuminuria.[73]
- Eye care: Practitioners and patients do not strictly follow the recommendation for eye examinations by ophthalmologists.[76] Effective treatments can prevent complications from diabetic retinopathy.[77]
- Foot care: Half of diabetic patients do not follow foot-care recommendations.[78] Practitioners do not regularly examine patients' feet, but interventions with appropriate follow-up do reduce foot lesions.[79;80]

Cardiovascular risks

Heart disease and related complications are the most common cause of death among patients with diabetes.[81] These patients have increased rates of macrovascular complications: 2 to 6 times greater risk for coronary artery and cerebrovascular disease,[82] and 5 times greater risk for intermittent claudication and gangrene (amputations).

Hemoglobin A1c predicts coronary artery disease. For example, the coronary heart disease mortality rate in Type 2 diabetes is about double from the lower tertile (Hb A1c < 6%) to the middle tertile (Hb A1c 6%-7.9%).[83] The majority of excessive health care and hospital drug costs are associated with cardiovascular disease.[84]

Smoking rates among diabetes patients are about the same as in the general population; just as in the general population, smoking greatly increases the risk of heart disease.[85;86] Cardiovascular risks are synergistically increased if patients smoke and have elevated cholesterol levels. The Scandinavian Simvastatin Survival Study showed that coronary deaths and nonfatal heart attacks were reduced by 54% in patients with diabetes, as compared to a 32% reduction in nondiabetic patients.[87;88] Statins lowered elevated LDL cholesterol in patients with diabetes and coronary artery disease and reduced cardiac events by 57% and mortality by 25%.[89] Thus, lowering hemoglobin A1c and cholesterol as much as possible reduces cardiovascular risk in patients with diabetes. Practitioners also should carefully consider how to treat heart disease and hypertension in patients with diabetes because some medications decrease insulin sensitivity (Propranolol, Metoprolol, Atenolol, hydrochlorothiazide, Verapamil, and furosemide), while others increase it (Doxazosin, Prazosin, Captopril, and Diltiazem).

Primary and secondary cardiovascular risk reduction is an emerging field in diabetic care. Primary preventive approaches may include using low-dose aspirin (in patients without proliferative retinopathy), folic acid (1 gram/day), and vitamin E (800 IU/per day).[90-93] Following an myocardial infarction, secondary prevention involves the use of intensive insulin therapy as opposed to standard care.[94] At a 3.4-year follow-up, intensive insulin therapy had a 33% opposed to a 44% mortality rate in standard care—a risk reduction of 25%.[89] Patients without prior cardiac history or insulin use had a mortality risk reduction of 58% and 52% during hospitalization and at one year, respectively.

E. Factors Hindering and Facilitating Self-care

Both individual and systemic factors can hinder or facilitate self-care of diabetes. (The role of supports and barriers in the self-care of diabetes was first addressed in Chapter 5 of *Beyond Advice: Becoming a Motivational Practitioner.*)

Depression

Depression may negatively impact patients in terms of caring for their diabetes, thus worsening glycemic control and increasing the likelihood of complications.[95] When patients experience such deterioration, you should consider depression in the differential diagnosis. Depression may be up to three times more common in adults with diabetes than in the general population; 20%-30% of adults with diabetes report depressive symptoms, and 14% are clinically depressed.[96] Unfortunately, it is often underdiagnosed in adults with diabetes.[97] Thus, the early detection of depression may help patients improve their glycemic control and prevent complications from neglect, such as failing to provide appropriate foot care.

Patient self-care skills

Practitioners are well advised to assess whether patients have the specific skills to take care of their diabetes.[37] Patient self-efficacy and expectations predict adherence to the recommendations for both types of diabetes.[42] Specific diabetic problem-solving skills are as strong a predictor of adequate glucose monitoring, exercise, and self-care as are other psychosocial variables.[44] Even when practitioners instruct patients about self-care skills, patients may develop the necessary skills but still not adhere to the recommendations. In many instances, patients already have related skills that they can apply to diabetes, but they do not use them consistently. Thus, practitioners should be aware that patients who are knowledgeable and skillful in self-care may still lack the motivation to adhere to recommendations over time.

Patient activation

Nonmedical staff can activate patients to enhance their self-care of diabetes. In one study, nonmedical staff spent about 20 minutes with patients preparing them for a visit with their physician. The staff reviewed medical charts with patients and encouraged them to ask questions and negotiate about treatment options. These patients lowered their hemoglobin A1c and reported less functional limitations, compared to the group of patients receiving routine care.[98]

Patient motivation

A randomized control study of comprehensive versus routine diabetic education for Type II diabetics (predominantly black and female) demonstrated that the comprehensive program significantly improved self-care skills (glucose testing, insulin-taking procedures, and reduced caloric intake), glycemic control, and other risk factors (e.g., blood pressure at 6-14 months follow-up) when compared to the routine program.[37;99] In contrast, another study on a weight reduction program in Type II diabetes showed that the intensive program helped patients lose more weight initially than the routine care group, but at one year, there was no difference between the two groups.[100]

With regard to using motivational interventions, four studies improved glycemic control when skills training with specific feedback was added to didactic education programs;[99;101-103] consequently, improved glycemic control was maintained for up to 2 years of follow-up.[104] Specific feedback is one of many motivational interventions that may help patients maintain change. Regrettably, many studies do not provide sufficient details about the extent to which they use different behavioral approaches. Thus, it is difficult to make meaningful comparisons between studies to help select interventions for individual patients.

Furthermore, most studies about diabetes have high attrition rates, which limits the generalizability of their findings to the population at large. The low participation and moderate attrition rates in many of these studies highlight a significant clinical issue: how to engage reluctant patients in programs that suit their disposition and needs. To take better care of their diabetes, patients need assistance in how to motivate or empower themselves to change.[43]

MOVING ON

Many factors affect patient outcomes. While you can educate patients to increase their knowledge and skills about diabetes, this alone does not necessarily improve patient adherence. Chapter 6b describes how you can motivate self-care of diabetes and improve patient outcomes.

Web Sites for Patients and Practitioners
A. Professional Resources
Medline plus health information about diabetes:
http://www.nlm.nih.gov/medlineplus/diabetes.html This site provides a master list of Web sites.
Health Finder (enter diabetes as a search): www.healthfinder.gov This site provides an abundance of information.
American Diabetes Association www.diabetes.org/Diabetes/: Clinical Practice Recommendations 1998 Report of the Expert Committee on the Diagnosis and Classification of Diabetes Mellitus: http://www.diabetes.org/Diabetescare/supplement198/S5.htm On page 19 of this report, the ADA suggests screening of individuals 45 and above, and if normal, repeating every three years.
Journal of the American Diabetes Association: www.diabetes.org/Diabetes/
Canadian Diabetes Association www.diabetes.ca/
U.S. Prevention Task Force Guidelines:
http://text.nlm.nih.gov/ftrs/directBrowse.pl?dbName=cps&href=CH19&t=979140827
The report does not support the ADA recommendation listed above, given the current level of evidence.
Health Care Financing Administration: http://www.hcfa.gov/quality/3r.htm This site contains a compendium of best practices by clicking on the links below:
       Introduction and Acknowledgments
       Section One: Improving Clinical Effectiveness
       Section Two: Federally Funded Diabetes Quality Improvement Projects
       Section Three: Worksite and Community-based Quality Improvement Projects
       Section Four: Bibliography—Clinical Efficacy
       Section Five: Appendix—Article Review Form
Section four has a list of good references.
CDC Division of Diabetes: http://www.cdc.gov/diabetes Call toll-free 1-877-CDC-DIAB (232-3422) or visit their Web site for CDC publications and products about diabetes (PDF files using Adobe Acrobat—one copy per person or a maximum of 50 per site) or use the a CDC order card (send one in per patient). Publication numbers are listed below. Their Web site is:
http://www.cdc.gov/diabetes/pubs/pubs.htm
0995114   Building Understanding to Prevent and Control Diabetes among Hispanics/Latinos
0994994   Diabetes at a Glance, 1999
0995586   Diabetes Surveillance, 1997
0996251   Division of Publication Request Post Card
0996013   Division Address/Telephone File Card, 2x3-inch

0995129	National Diabetes Fact Sheet (English)
0995875	National Diabetes Fact Sheet (Spanish)
0995490	National Hispanic/Latino Diabetes Initiative for Action Recommendations Report
0995777	National Hispanic/Latino Report: CDC Response
0995276	Take Charge of Your Diabetes (English, Bound)
0994292	Take Charge of Your Diabetes (English, Camera-Ready)
0995479	Take Charge of Your Diabetes (Spanish, Bound)
0995398	Take Charge of Your Diabetes (Spanish, Camera-Ready)
0996146	The Economics of Diabetes Mellitus: An Annotated Bibliography

NIDDK—National Institute of Diabetes and Digestive and Kidney Diseases: This is a Web site with many PDF files that you can print up and use in your programs. Some examples are; "Feet Can Last a Lifetime": www.niddk.nih.gov/health/diabetes/feet/feet2/index.htm

"Diabetes Nutrition Series": www.niddk.nih.gov/health/diabetes/pubs/nutritn/index.htm You can download a PDF file or order easy-to-read brochures/pamphlets in both Spanish and English.

"Clinical Guidelines for Nutrition & Obesity": www.niddk.nih.gov/health/nutrit/nutrit.htm This site also has links to numerous sites for people with diabetes who have a weight problem or need help with an exercise program. You can print these files (most are in PDF format) and if you have a color printer you can dress them up for handouts. Once you have reached that site you can go into the link files: for example, "You Can Control Your Weight As You Quit Smoking," "Physical Activity and Weight Control," "Weight Loss for Life," "Sisters Together: Move More, Eat Better."

"Improving Health Tips for African American Men & Women": www.niddk.nih.gov/health/nutrit/pubs/wintips/index.htm

"Walking…A Step in the Right Direction":www.niddk.nih.gov/health/nutrit/pubs/walking.htm

"Release of Clinical Guidelines to Identify, Evaluate and Treat Overweight and Obesity in Adults": www.niddk.nih.gov/health/nutrit/nutrit.htm This link to NHLBI (National Heart, Lung and Blood Institute) has a downloadable, large PDF file. If you have the time to print it, it would save you some costs. Or, the direct site where you can order is: www.nhlbi.gov/guidelines/obesity/ob_gdlns.htm

Clinician National Forum for Underserved Populations: http://cnf.org/diabetes/diabetes.htm This Web site describes the work of a national diabetes collaborative that uses quality improvement methods and population-based approaches to enhance the care of diabetes. It lists a site for evidence-based approaches and addresses the issue of re-engineering the patient visit.

The Merck Manual: www.merck.com/pubs/mmanual Search "diabetes mellitus" for further information. Articles/chapters can be printed from the computer.

Ask NOAH About Diabetes: www.noahcuny.edu/diabetes/diabetes.html This Web site offers many links to various topics regarding diabetes. Most of these are verified sites; some were found not to exist anymore. Topics include: The Basics on Diabetes; Complications and Related Concerns; Care and Treatment; and Diabetes Resources.

L.E.A.P. (Lower Extremity Amputation Prevention Program): http://www.bphc.hrsa.dhhs.gov/leap/def.htm This site has information regarding this program. Patients can call the 1-800-275-4772 number and receive a free monofilament and foot screening guide to use at home (The Feet Can Last A Lifetime information has the 5-site foot screen form that is consistent with HCFA, NIDDK, and ADA recommendations). This site is being updated and will have the training brochure in multiple languages when it is completed. Clinics can call and get a maximum of 50 copies. Make sure you utilize these screening guides and coordinate the "Feet Can Last A Lifetime" program through NIDDK (which is being updated). These two programs complement each other.

Doctor's Guide to Diabetes Information & Resources:
http://www.pslgroup.com/DIABETES.HTM This site contains the latest medical news and information for patients or friends/parents of patients diagnosed with diabetes and diabetes-related disorders. They have links on "Medical News and Alerts"; "Diabetes Information"; "Discussion Groups and Newsgroups" and "Other Related Sites." There is also a signup if you want them to e-mail you on any changes to that information.

Joslin Diabetes Center: www.joslin.harvard.edu/;This is a site for both professional and lay audiences.

Juvenile Diabetes Foundation (JDF) International: www.jdf.org/ This site focuses on the research aspects of curing diabetes

Diabetes.com: Latest Diabetes Information & Community: www.diabetes.com/

The Diabetes Monitor: www.diabetesmonitor.com/ This site monitors what is going on in cyberspace on diabetes.

Diabetes: Drug Information Center: www.pharminfo.com/disease/diabetes/diab_info.html

Rick Mendosa's Diabetes Directory: www.mendosa.com/diabetes.htm

Improving Cardiovascular Health in African Americans:
www.nhlbi.nih.gov/health/public/heart/other/chdblack/index.htm This site is under the National Heart, Lung and Blood Institute. You can order (there is a cost) or download from the PDF file. This is a great way to get information on those issues with diabetes.

National Coalition for Promoting Physical Activity: www.ncppa.org or call 1-317-637-0349. The Month of May is Physical Fitness and Sports Month. Utilize this guide to get your programs going in May to help promote good fitness and exercise with your clients who have diabetes.

Medscape: http://www.diabetes.medscape.com or http://www.medscape.com This site is where you can sign up for free weekly updates on chronic diseases and health issues. It is a great site and will send disease-specific articles right to your e-mail. You then have the ability to either print or send them to someone else.

B. Patient Resources

On-Line Diabetes Resources: www.diabetesmonitor.com/mag.htm or www.diabetesmonitor.com/nonengl.htm This Web site has both English and non-English Web links available. They cover everything from *Diabetic Cooking* magazine to books you can browse through on the Internet relating to diabetes. The non-English site has pharmaceutical companies with Web sites in different languages, as well as newsletters and articles in Spanish. There is also a link on the front page that has additional languages.

Diabetes on About.com: www.diabetes.about.com/health/diabetes/mbody.htm This provides a guide to more than 700 Web sites.

The Healing Handbook for Persons with Diabetes:
www.ummed.edu/dept/diabetes/handbook/toc.htm Ruth E Lundstrom, R.N., and Aldo A. Rossini, M.D., have written this book that is downloadable from this Web site. (You will have to print each chapter separately and the book is large.) You will see a disclaimer at the very back of the Chapter "Looking to the Future." This should be taken note of on all printed materials unless it is an educational piece specifically designed for patient education. Since this book is printable in chapter form, you could print only those chapters needed.

Diabetes and Your Feet: www.footcare4u.com/aodf/index.html This Web site has some good, easy-to-understand drawings and written information regarding foot complications with individuals who have diabetes. There are quite a few links, but the better information is located at the Treatments; Nerve Damage; Circulation Problems; Complications; and Self-Care sections.

America's Diabetes Health Record Passport: http://www.securitec.com/DHR.html They will send you examples of the passport at your request. This is not a free service, as the passports do cost, but they have a larger-quantity discount. Visit the Web site or call 1-800-783-2145.

The Diabetes Mall: http://www.diabetesnet.com This Web site offers a host of different links, such as newsroom, bookstore, diabetes facts, and stories on specific topics. You can also sign up for a free e-mail newsletter, but a warning—they ask for your phone number, age and other personal information. You can still sign up and leave them blank. The stories appear to be current with medical news. Remember, be careful on giving sites that have diagnostic information to patients—they may play doctor.

Multi-Ethnic Health care—Closing the Gap:
http://www.closing-the-gap.com/Departments/Centers/diabetes.html This site has information regarding diabetes, asthma and allergies, cancer, heart disease and a few other diseases. It is sponsored by Pfizer, which has a direct link. There is a free e-mail update you can sign up for, as well as information on diseases, cultural issues, practitioner's corner, and media corner with the latest news releases.

Diabetic Gourmet: http://www.diabeticgourmet.com This Web site has lots of good information, such as recipes; Diabetes 101 (basic diabetes information); topics and tips; shopping links and latest press releases about diabetes. There is a free newsletter you can sign up for by just completing the questions.

Diabetic Lifestyle: Online Magazine: http://www.diabetic-lifestyle.com/index.htm This is also a site with great recipes, as well as exercise tips, kids section, travel, and the latest diabetes health updates.

Diabetes Digest: http://www.diabetesdigest.com/ This site has a free online newsletter providing diabetes information for the patient and doctor. There are lots of items you can print up as well as health tips and recipes you can give to patients.

Diabetes Life Network: www.diabeteslife.net/pros/continue.html They have a continuing education section where you can link to other Web sites and receive information about continuing education efforts and diabetes information. The one link that is particularly good on this site is www.diabeteslife.net/kids/manual/index.html. This is a PDF file that can be printed and used with low-literacy educational programs. It is geared toward kids, but could be used in the same context with adults.

Diabetes Portal: www.diabetesportal.com
This Web site gives up-to-date developments in the care of diabetes through a network of additional Web sites. This site includes:
Diabetes Living: www.diabetesliving.com Covers the basics, diabetes management, parenting and children, complications, coping and what's new.
Diabetes Warehouse: www.diabeteswarehouse.com A shopping place for patients with diabetes.
Diabetes Station: www.DiabetesStation.org Provides Web broadcasts of recent developments.
Diabetes Portal provides site for recent research developments, including islet cell transplantation.

Eli Lilly and Company: http://diabetes.lilly.com Eli Lilly provides useful patient education materials. Their Web site contains quick, short informational pieces that complement their brochures and handouts. Their patient education materials include: Controlling Your Blood Sugar; Planning Your Meals; Stages of Care; Getting Started with Exercise; How to Manage Gestational Diabetes; Basic Facts About Diabetes; Managing Your Diabetes; and a Daily Meal Planning Guide. Check with your local pharmaceutical representative on getting one or more of these publications

MyDiabetes.com: www.mydiabetes.com You have to register to use this Web site.

Diabetes Well: www.diabeteswell.com This site provides online support for patients. A free 90-day period is offered.

Diabetic Cooking: www.DiabeticCooking.com This site provide tips for cooking.

Yahoo! Health & Diabetes: www.yahoo.com/Health/Diseases_and_Conditions/Diabetes/

NutritionU Columbia University: www.nutritionu.com You have to register to use this site and learn more about nutrition and diabetes.

Division of Nutritional Health and Services:
www.health.state.mo.us/NutritionServices/EastForHealth.html This site is from the main Department of Health's home page. A great place to print recipes and tips; they have program materials you can download. Make sure you go to the Missouri Nutrition Network section.

Fast Food Facts: www.childrenwithdiabetes.com/d_08_700.htm This site has information on calories and carbos of fast food. Print and give to your patients.

Dietary Guidelines for Americans: www.nalusda.gov/fnic/dga/dguide95.html This site has some great information you can print.

Diabetes Self-Management: Recipe Directory: www.diabetes-self-mgmt.com/dir_rec.html This site has some healthy recipes for your patients.

Sweetener Web Sites: These Web sites have recipes, exchange tables, and sweetener information. Check them all out and let your patients decide what works best for them.

> Equal—www.equal.com
> SweetOne—www.sweetone.com
> Sweet'N Low—www.sweetnlow.com

Novo Nordisk: www.novonordisk.com/educate/intro.asp Novo Nordisk has some great educational materials available by calling 1-800-727-6500 or visiting their Web site. (For large quantities, contact your local sales representative.)

Becton Dickinson: www.bd.com/diabetes/ Has some great educational materials as well, and you can order through their Web site. (BD will provide 25 free through their Web site. For additional copies, contact your local sales representative.)

Food Guide Pyramid: www.eatright.org/nfs/nfs0399sp.html This site is in Spanish.

Weight Management Techniques: www.eatright.org/nfs/nfs70.html

Preparing Nutritious Meals at Minimal Cost—U.S. Department of Agriculture:
www.usda.gov/cnpp/FoodPlans/TFP99/food$pdf.PDF
www.usda.gov/cnpp This is their main site with great links to additional information.

Reference List

1. Wang PH, Lau J, Chalmers TC. Meta-analysis of effect of intensive blood glucose control on late complications of type 1 diabetes. Lancet 1993;341: 1306-1309
2. Reichard P, Nilsson B-Y, Rosenquist U. The effect of long-term intensified insulin treatment on the development of micro-vascular complications of diabetes mellitus. New England Journal of Medicine 1993;329: 304-309

3. The Diabetes Control and Complications Trial Research Group. The relationship of glycemic exposure (HbA1c) to the risk of development and progression of retinopathy in the Diabetes Control and Complications Trail. Diabetes 1995;44: 968-983

4. Glasgow RE, Anderson BJ. Future directions for research on pediatric chronic disease management: Lessons from diabetes. Journal of Pediatric Psychology 1995;20: 389-402

5. The Diabetes Control and Complications Trial Research Group. The effect of intensive treatment of diabetes on the development and progression of long-term complications in insulin-dependent diabetes mellitus. New England Journal of Medicine 1993;329: 977-986

6. Ohkubo Y, Kishikawa H, Araki E, et al. Intensive insulin therapy prevents the progression of diabetic microvascular complications in Japanese patients with non-insulin-dependent diabetes mellitus: a randomized prospective 6-year study. Diabetes Research and Clinical Practice 1995;28: 103-117

7. Matthews DR, Cull CA, Stratton IM, et al. UKPDS 26: Sulphonylurea failure in non-insulin-dependent diabetic patients over six years. UK Prospective Diabetes Study (UKPDS) Group. Diabetic Medicine 1998;15: 297-303

8. UK Prospective Diabetes Study (UKPDS). Tight blood pressure control and risk of macrovascular and microvascular complications in type 2 diabetes: UKPDS 38. British Medical Journal 1998;317: 703-713

9. UK Prospective Diabetes Study (UKPDS). Efficacy of atenolol and captopril in reducing risk of macrovascular and microvascular complications in type 2 diabetes: UKPDS 39. British Medical Journal 1998;317: 713-720

10. UK Prospective Diabetes Study (UKPDS). Cost effectiveness analysis of improved blood pressure control in hypertensive patients with type 2 diabetes: UKPDS 40. British Medical Journal 1998;317: 720-726

11. Mogenson CE. Combined high blood pressure and glucose in type 2 diabetes: double jeopardy; British trial shows clear effects of treatment, especially blood pressure reduction. British Medical Journal 1998;317: 693-694

12. Nathan DM. Some answers, more controversy, from UKPDS. United Kingdom Prospective Diabetes Study [comment]. Lancet 1998;352: 832-833

13. UK Prospective Diabetes Study (UKPDS). Effect of intensive blood-glucose control with metformin on complications in overweight patients with type 2 diabetes (UKPDS 34). UK Prospective Diabetes Study (UKPDS) Group [see comments]. Lancet 1998;352: 854-865

14. The Diabetes Control and Complications Trial Research Group. Lifetime benefits and costs of intensive therapy as practiced in the diabetes control and complications trial. JAMA 1996;276: 1409-1415

15. Rubin RJ, Altman WM, Mendelson DN. Health care expenditures for people with diabetes mellitus. Journal of Clinical Endocrinology & Metabolism 1994;78: 809A-809F

16. O'Connor PJ, Rush WA, Peterson J, et al. Continuous quality improvement can improve glycemic control for HMO patients with diabetes. Archives of Family Medicine 1996;5: 502-506

17. American Diabetes Association. Medical management of non-insulin-dependent (Type II) diabetes. 3 ed. USA: American Diabetes Assoc.; 1994

18. American Diabetes Association. Standards of medical care for patients with diabetes mellitus. Diabetes Care 1995;18: 8-23

19. American Diabetes Association. Medical management of insulin-dependent (Type I) diabetes. 2 ed. USA: American Diabetes Assoc.; 1994

20. Clark C, Lee A. Prevention and treatment of the complications of diabetes mellitus. The New England Journal of Medicine 1995;332(18): 1208-1217

21. Kerr CP. Improving outcomes in diabetes: A review of the outpatient care of NIDDM patients. Journal of Family Practice 1995;40: 63-75

22. Coonrod BA, Betschart J, Harris MI. Frequency and determinants of diabetes patient education among adults in the U.S. population. Diabetes Care 1994;17: 852-858

23. Etzwiler DD. Diabetes translation: A blueprint for the future. Diabetes Care 1994;17: 1-4

24. American Diabetes Association. Nutrition recommendations and principles for people with diabetes mellitus. Diabetes Care 1996;19: S16-S19

25. Harris MI, Eastman RC, Siebert C. The DCCT and medical care for diabetes in the U.S. Diabetes Care 1994;17: 761-764

26. Marrero DG. Current effectiveness of diabetes health care in the U.S. Diabetes Review 1994;2: 292-309

27. Anderson RM, Fitzgerald JT, Funnell MM, et al. Evaluation of an activated patient diabetes education newsletter. Diabetes Educator 1994;20: 29-34

28. Glasgow RE, McCaul KD, Schafer LC. Self-care behaviors and glycemic control in Type I diabetes. Journal of Chronic Diseases 1987;40: 399-412

29. Wilson W, Ary DV, Biglan A, et al. Psychosocial predictors of self-care behaviors (compliance) and glycemic control in non-insulin dependent diabetes mellitus. Diabetes Care 1986;9: 614-622

30. Johnson SB, Silverstein J, Rosenbloom AR, et al. Assessing daily management in childhood diabetes. Health Psychology 1986;5: 545-564

31. Orme CM, Binik YM. Consistency of adherence across regimen demands. Health Psychology 1989;8: 27-43

32. Irvine A. Self care behaviors in a rural population with diabetes. Patient Education and Counseling 1989;13: 3-13

33. Ary DV, Toobert D, Wilson W, et al. Patient perspective on factors contributing to nonadherence to diabetes regimens. Diabetes Care 1986;9: 168-172

34. House WC, Pendleton L, Parker L. Patients' versus physicians' attributions of reasons for diabetic patients' noncompliance with diet. Diabetes Care 1986;9: 434

35. Diehl AK, Bauer RL, Sugarek NJ. Correlates of medical compliance in non-insulin diabetes mellitus. Southern Medical Journal 1987;80: 332-335

36. Mazzuca SA. Does patient education in chronic disease have therapeutic value? Journal of Chronic Disease 1982;35: 521-529

37. Glasgow R. Compliance to diabetes regimens: Conceptualization, complexity, and determinants. In: Cramer JA, Spilker B, eds. Patient compliance in medical practice and clinical trials 1 ed. New York: Raven Press; 1991:209-224

38. Ley P. Psychological studies of doctor-patient communication. In: S. Rachman S. (Ed.). Contributions to medical psychology 1977; 9-42

39. Mazzuca SA, Weinberger M, Kurpius DJ, et al. Clinician communication associated with diabetic patients' comprehension of their therapeutic regimen. Diabetes Care 1983;6: 347-350

40. Goodall T, Halford WK. Self-management of diabetes mellitus: A critical review. Health Psychology 1991;10(1): 1-8

41. Watkins JD, Williams TF, Martin DA, et al. A study of diabetic patients at home. American Journal of Public Health 1967;57: 452-459

42. McCaul KD, Glasgow RE, Schafer LC. Diabetes regimen behaviors: Predicting adherence. Medical Care 1987;25: 868-881

43. Anderson RM, Funnell MM, Butler PM, et al. Patient empowerment: Results of a randomized controlled trial. Diabetes Care 1995;18: 943-949

44. Toobert DJ, Glasgow RE. Problem solving and diabetes self-care. Journal of Behavioral Medicine 1991;14: 71-86

45. Clement S. Diabetes self-management education. Diabetes Care 1995;18: 1204-1214

46. Glasgow RE, Toobert DJ, Hampson SE. Effects of a brief office-based intervention to facilitate diabetes dietary self-management. Diabetes Care 1996;19: 835-842

47. Kirkman MS, Weinberger M, Landsman PB, et al. A telephone-delivered intervention for patients with NIDDM: Effect on coronary risk factors. Diabetes Care 1994;17: 840-846

48. Wasson J, Gaudette C, Whaley F, et al. Telephone care as a substitute for routine clinic follow-up. JAMA 1992;267: 1788-1793

49. Christensen NK, Terry RD, Wyatt S, et al. Quantitative assessment of dietary adherence in patients with insulin-dependent diabetes mellitus. Diabetes Care 1983;6: 245-250

50. Anderson RM, Nowacek G, Richards F. Influencing the personal meaning of diabetes: Research and practice. Diabetes Educator 1988;14: 297-302

51. Johnson SB. Regimen adherence: Roles and responsibilities of health care providers. Diabetes Spectrum 1993;6(3): 204-205

52. Tinker LF, Heins JM, Holler H. Commentary and translation: 1994 nutrition recommendations for diabetes. Diabetes Spectrum 1994;7: 225-230

53. Wing RR, Epstein LH, Nowalk MP, et al. Does self-monitoring of blood glucose levels improve dietary compliance for obese patients with Type II diabetes? The American Journal of Medicine 1986;81: 830-835

54. Wing RR, Marcus MD, Epstein LH, et al. Type II diabetic subjects lose less weight than their overweight non-diabetic spouses. Diabetes Care 1987;10: 563-566

55. Wing RR. Improving weight loss and maintenance in patients with diabetes. In: Anderson BJ, Rubin RR, eds. Practical psychology for diabetes clinicians. Alexandria, VA: American Diabetes Assoc.; 1996:113-120

56. Marcus BH, Eaton CA, Rossi JS, et al. Self-efficacy, decision making, and stages of change: An integrative model of physical exercise. Journal of Applied Social Psychology 1994;24(6): 489-508

57. Rossi JS, Rossi SR, Velicer WF, et al. Motivational readiness to control weight: The transtheoretical model of behavior change. In: Allison DB, ed. Methods for assessment of eating behaviors and weight related problems. Newbury Park, CA: Sage Publications; 1993:

58. Pate RR, Pratt M, Blair SN, et al. Physical activity and public health. A recommendation from the Centers for Disease Control and Prevention and the American College of Sports Medicine [see comments]. JAMA 1995;273: 402-407

59. Wing RR, Epstein LH, Paternostro-Bayles M, et al. Exercise in a behavioural weight control programme for obese patients with Type 2 (non-insulin-dependent) diabetes. Diabetologia 1988;31: 902-909

60. Wilson DP, Endres RK. Compliance with blood glucose monitoring in children with Type I diabetes mellitus. Journal of Pediatrics 1986;108: 1022-1024

61. Mazze RS, Pasmantier R, Murphy JA, et al. Self-monitoring of capillary blood glucose: Changing the performance of individuals with diabetes. Diabetes Care 1985;8: 207-213

62. Gonder-Frederick LA, Julian DM, Cox DJ, et al. Self-measurement of blood glucose: Accuracy of self-reported data and adherence to recommended regimen. Diabetes Care 1988;11: 579-585

63. Davidson MB. Futility of self-monitoring of blood glucose without algorithms for adjusting insulin doses. Diabetes Care 1986;9: 209-210

64. Cohen S, Wills TA. Stress, social support and the buffering hypothesis. Psychological Bulletin 1985;98: 310-357

65. Groggel GC. Diabetic nephropathy. Archives of Family Medicine 1996;5: 513-520

66. Poirier SJ. Preserving the diabetic kidney. Journal of Family Practice 1998;46: 21-27

67. Lewis EJ, Hunsicker LG, Bain RP, et al. The effect of angiotensin-converting-enzyme inhibition on diabetic nephropathy. The Collaborative Study Group. New England Journal of Medicine 1993;329: 1456-1462

68. Ravid M, Savin H, Jutrin I, et al. Long-term stabilizing effect of angiotensin-converting enzyme inhibition on plasma creatinine and on proteinuria in normotensive Type II diabetic patients. Annals of Internal Medicine 1993;118: 577-581

69. Bennett PH, Haffner S, Kasiske BL, et al. Screening and management of microalbuminuria in patients with diabetes mellitus: Recommendations to the Scientific Advisory Board of the National Kidney Foundation from an ad hoc committee of the Council on Diabetes Mellitus of the National Kidney Foundation. American Journal of Kidney Diseases 1995;25: 107-112

70. Davidson MB. Treating microalbuminuria: Are ACE inhibitors the answer? Practical Diabetology 1993;June: 10-13

71. Nelson RG, Knowler WC, Pettitt DJ, et al. Assessment of risk of overt nephropathy in diabetic patients from albumin excretion in untimed urine specimens. Archives of Internal Medicine 1991;151: 1761-1765

72. Alzaid AA. Microalbuminuria in patients with NIDDM: An overview. Diabetes Care 1996;19: 79-89

73. Mogensen CE. Microalbuminuria predicts clinical proteinuria and early mortality in maturity-onset diabetes. New England Journal of Medicine 1984;310: 356-360

74. Niskanen LK, Penttila I, Parviainen M, et al. Evolution, risk factors, and prognostic implications of albuminuria in NIDDM. Diabetes Care 1996;19: 486-493

75. DeFronzo RA. Diabetic nephropathy: Etiologic and therapeutic considerations. Diabetes Metabolism Review 1995;3: 510-564

76. Kraft SK, Marrero DG, Lazaridis EN, et al. Primary care physicians' practice patterns and diabetic retinopathy. Current levels of care. Archives of Family Medicine 1997;6: 29-37

77. Clinical Trials Branch, National Eye Institute. How Effective Are Treatments for Diabetic Retinopathy. JAMA 1993;269(10): 1290-1277

78. Gross A.M. A behavioral approach to the compliance problems of young diabetics. Journal of Compliance in Health Care 1987;2: 7-21

79. Litzelman DK, Slemenda CW, Langefeld CD, et al. Reduction of lower extremity clinical abnormalities in patients with non-insulin-dependent diabetes mellitus. A randomized, controlled trial. Annals of Internal Medicine 1993;119: 36-41

80. Echman M, Greenfield S, Mackey W, et al. Foot Infections in Diabetic Patients: Decisions and cost effectiveness analyses. JAMA 1995;273(9): 712-723

81. Brownson RC, Remington PL, Davis JR. Chronic disease epidemiology and control. Baltimore, MD: Port City Press; 1993

82. Yoshinari M, Kaku R, Iwase M, et al. Development of ischemic stroke in normotensive and hypertensive diabetic patients with or without antihypertensive treatment: An 8-year followup study. Journal of Diabetes & its Complications 1997;11: 9-14

83. Kuusisto J, Mykkanen L, Pyorala K, et al. NIDDM and its metabolic control predict coronary heart disease in elderly subjects. Diabetes 1994;43: 960-967

84. Glauber H, Brown J. Impact of cardiovascular disease on health care utilization in a defined diabetic population. Journal of Clinical Epidemiology 1994;47: 1133-1142

85. Fisher EB, Jr., Arfken CL, Heins JM, et al. Acceptance of diabetes regimens in adults. In: Gochman DS, ed. Handbook of health behavior research II: Provider determinants. New York: Plenum Press; 1997:189-212

86. Haire-Joshu D. Smoking, cessation, and the diabetes health care team. Diabetes Educator 1991;17: 54-64

87. Pyorala, K., Pedersen, T. R., and Kjekshus, J. The effect of cholesterol lowering with simvastatin on coronary events in diabetic patients with coronary heart disease. Diabetes 44[Suppl. 1], 35A. 1995.

88. Kjekshus J, Pedersen TR. Reducing the risk of coronary events: Evidence from the Scandinavian Simvastatin Survival Study (4S). The American Journal of Cardiology 1995;76: 64c-68c

89. Hafner SM. Management of dyslipidemia in adults with diabetes. Diabetes Care 1998;21: 160-178

90. Stampfer MJ, Rimm EB. Folate and cardiovascular disease: Why we need a trial now. JAMA 1996;275: 1929-1930

91. Rimm EB, Willett WC, Hu FB, et al. Folate and vitamin B6 from diet and supplements in relation to risk of coronary heart disease among women. JAMA 1998;279: 359-364

92. Gazis A, Page S, Cockcroft J. Vitamin E and cardiovascular protection in diabetes. BMJ 1997;314: 1845-1846

93. Stephens NG, Parsons A, Schofield PM, et al. Randomised controlled trial of vitamin E in patients with coronary disease: Cambridge Heart Antioxidant Study (CHAOS). Lancet 1996;347: 781-786

94. Malmberg K, Ryden L, Efendic S, et al. Randomized trial of insulin-glucose infusion followed by subcutaneous insulin treatment in diabetic patients with acute myocardial infarction (DIGAMI study): Effects on mortality at 1 year. Journal of the American College of Cardiology 1995;26: 57-65

95. Lustman PJ, Griffith LS, Gavard JA, et al. Depression in adults with diabetes. Diabetes Care 1992;15: 1631-1639

96. Gavard JA, Lustman PJ, Clouse RE. Prevalence of depression in adults with diabetes: An epidemiological evaluation. Diabetes Care 1993;16: 1167-1178

97. Lustman PJ, Griffith LS, Clouse RE. Recognizing and managing depression in patients with diabetes. In: Anderson BJ, Rubin RR, eds. Practical psychology for diabetes clinicians. Alexandria, VA: American Diabetes Assoc.; 1996:143-154

98. Greenfield S, Kaplan SH, Ware JE, Jr., et al. Patients' participation in medical care: Effects on blood sugar control and quality of life in diabetes. Journal of General Internal Medicine 1988;3: 448-457

99. Mazzuca SA, Moorman NH, Wheeler M. The diabetes education study: A controlled trial of the effects of diabetes patient education. Diabetes Care 1986;9: 1-10

100. Wing RR, Epstein LH, Nowalk MP, et al. Behavior change, weight loss and physiological improvements in Type II diabetic patients. Journal of Consulting and Clinical Psychology 1985;53: 111-122

101. Buysschaert M, Lepair-Gadiseuz N, Weil R, et al. Effect of an in-patient education programme upon the knowledge, behaviour and glycaemic control of insulin-dependent diabetic patients. Diabete and Metabolisme 1987;13: 31-36

102. McCulloch DK, Mitchell RD, Ambler J, et al. Influence of imaginative teaching of diet on compliance and metabolic control in insulin dependent diabetes. British Medical Journal 1983;28: 1858-1861

103. Wise PH, Dowlatshahi DC, Farrant S, et al. Effect of computer-based learning on diabetes knowledge and control. Diabetes Care 1986;9: 504-508

104. Vinicor F, Cohen SJ, Mazzuca SA, et al. Diabeds: A randomized trial of the effects of physician and/or patient education on diabetes patient outcomes. Journal of Chronic Disease 1987;40: 345-356

CHAPTER 6b

FACILITATING SELF-CARE OF DIABETES

FOR REFLECTION

How can you help patients adhere to multiple recommendations in order to:
- *Lower hemoglobin A1c as much as possible?*
- *Reduce the rate of diabetic complications?*
- *Slow the deterioration rate of diabetic complications?*
- *Lessen the impact of complications when they occur?*

OVERVIEW

This chapter describes how you can develop individualized interventions to help patients take better care of their diabetes. You can negotiate with patients about whether and how to adhere to the diabetic guidelines and thereby work toward reducing Hb A1c levels, the complication rates, and the impact of those complications.

FACILITATING SELF-CARE OF DIABETES

To learn new skills in addressing multiple agendas, work with a patient who has diabetes. Refer to Chapter 4b or 5b to find an increased range of possibilities for using the six-step approach to its full advantage.

STEP 1: BUILDING PARTNERSHIPS

Communication Skills for Developing Empathy	
Use open-ended questions	*"Tell me how diabetes interferes with enjoying life."*
Use reflective listening	*"So, you enjoy eating doughnuts and..."*
Paraphrase	*"You know how to control your diabetes, but other things seem to have a higher priority than your diabetes."*
Validate feelings	*"So, sometimes you do feel a little guilty about eating doughnuts."*
Normalize behaviors	*"It's quite common for people not to keep to their diet all of the time."*
Affirm strengths	*"But you take your medication regularly and watch your diet most of the time."*
Use probing questions	*"What would it take for you to keep more on top of your diabetes?"*

Relational Skills
Put the patient in the one-up position: *"What might convince you that you are at risk of developing diabetic complications?"* *"What might convince you to take better control of your diabetes?"*   *"You know what to do, but what do you think is stopping you from doing it?"*
Take the one-down position with a patient: *"I am not sure what it would take to convince you about your risk of developing complications."* *"I'm not sure what would convince you to take better control of your diabetes."*
Clarifying Roles
Clarify your prevention role: *"Diabetes can damage your health even when you feel well and before you get any symptoms. Can I help keep you from letting diabetes damage your health?"*   Clarify your motivational role: *"There is a lot you can do to stop diabetes from damaging your health, particularly when you're feeling so well. Can I help you so you can take better care of your diabetes?"*

Clarifying Responsibility
"I'll tell you what I know about the risk of developing diabetic complications (practitioner's responsibility), but we may still see the benefits and risks of good diabetic control differently. We can work together to understand our differences (a shared responsibility). I can help you increase your motivation to change (practitioner's responsibility), but it is up to you whether you can keep your hemoglobin A1c in the normal range (patient's responsibility)."

STEP 2: NEGOTIATING AN AGENDA

A. Prevention-focused Approach[a]

Consent-gaining, Direct Questions
"I'd like to check on whether there is anything you can do to improve your diabetes. Is that all right?" [Let patient respond.] You can then ask some direct questions. Opened-ended questions: *"There are several things we could discuss about diabetes. What would you like to talk about?"* [Ask one or more of the following questions.] *"How are you doing with the diet?"* *"What's it like for you to live with diabetes?"* *"What are you doing to control your blood glucose levels?"* *"How does your living with diabetes affect your family?"* Or, *"I would like to talk about whether you are interested in doing anything more to deal with your diabetes. Is that all right?"* [Let patient respond.] You can then ask, *"Is there anything that you want to discuss?"* Focused, open-ended questions: *"In what ways does your busy life cause difficulties in caring for your diabetes?"* *"How does your family help you deal with the care of your diabetes?"* Closed-ended questions: *"Do you take your tablets?"* *"Do you keep to your diet?"* *"Do you check your blood glucose regularly?"*

Leading Questions
"I'd like to ask about the kinds of food you like to eat. Do you have a favorite food that you know you shouldn't eat?" *"What do you like to eat when you go out with friends?"* *"How often do you forget to take your tablets?"*
Prefacing Statements
"It is difficult to deal with all the diabetic recommendations. What do you find most difficult to deal with?"

B. Problem-focused Approach

Prefacing Statements Followed by Leading Questions
"Your hemoglobin A1c is 11.8. What you do understand about that result?"   *"Most patients find it difficult to remember to take their tablets every day, particularly when they feel well. How often do you forget to take your tablets?"*   *"Most patients find it difficult to keep to the diabetic diet. What do you find most difficult or inconvenient about this diet?"*   *"Many patients get fed up with checking their blood glucose levels. What do you find is most inconvenient about checking your sugar levels?"*   Normalizing and validating comments: *"Patients find it difficult to keep to the diabetic diet and to lose weight. What do you find difficult about keeping to a diet and losing weight?"*   Preparing patients for nonpharmacological interventions [Type II diabetes]: *"We need to talk about either adding another drug, using insulin injections, or losing weight. Let me explain. If you lose weight, you might be able to lower your blood glucose to a point where you won't need to take another tablet or use insulin injections. Perhaps we can talk about your diet and weight reduction as a way to avoid adding another tablet or using insulin injections."* [Let patient respond.]   Comments that explore patients' concerns about consequences: *"Have you any concerns about having hypoglycemic episodes if we try to keep your blood glucose at normal levels?"*

Exploratory Questions
Open-ended, linear questions: *"How has your infection affected your blood glucose levels?"*   *"How have your concerns about angina affected what you do in dealing with your diabetes?"*   Closed-ended, linear questions: *"Has the infection affected your appetite?"*   *"Has your illness affected how often you check your blood sugar?"*   *"Have your symptoms made you feel less inclined to keep on top of your diabetes?"*   [Let patient respond.]   Circular questions: *"What concerns does your spouse have about how diabetes affects your health? What does your spouse think about how you are dealing with your diabetes?"*

STEP 3: ASSESSING RESISTANCE AND MOTIVATION

Readiness to Change
"Where are you in terms of dealing with (diabetic diet, weight reduction goals, glucose monitoring, exercise)?" [You can select one of the following three questions, or sequence them according to your impression of the patient.]   *"Are you not really thinking about changing?"*   *"Are you thinking about it?"*   *"Are you willing to make a change?"*

Providing Stage-specific Rationale and Gaining Consent to Use the Decision Balance
Precontemplation: *"You just told me that you are not thinking about changing your diet or losing weight. We could do a decision balance together because it could help both of us better understand why you want to continue as you are. Is that okay?"*
Contemplation: *"You told me how much you struggle with trying to keep to your diet and lose weight. We could do a decision balance together because it could help you think more seriously about change."*
Preparation: *"You're seriously thinking about keeping to your diet better and losing weight. We could do a decision balance together because it could help motivate you to set a date to change."*
Action: *"You seem ready to set a date to change. We could do a decision balance together because it could help prevent you relapsing to your old ways."*

Showing the Decision Balance to the Patient	
"Let me show you what a decision balance looks like. As we use the decision balance, it can help you better understand your reasons to stay the same and your reasons to lose weight and go on a diet. But first [pointing to the top middle column]*, I would like you to list as many benefits as possible from eating what you like. I would like to make a note of what you say. Is that okay? You can keep this decision balance to use when you go home if you like."* You can ask one or more of the following questions from each quadrant.	
Reasons to Stay the Same	Reasons to Change
Benefits of eating anything *"What are the benefits of eating what you want, as opposed to sticking to the diabetic diet? Does eating food benefit you in other ways; for example, to relax or relieve stress?"* [Let patient respond.] *"And what else?"*	Concerns about eating anything *"What concerns you about eating what you want?"* [Pause and let patient respond.] *"How might diabetic complications interfere with any other parts of your life?"* [Pause and let patient respond.] *"What, if anything, concerns you about not having a normal Hb A1c?"*
Concerns about dieting and weight loss *"What concerns you about keeping to the diabetic diet?"* *"What, if anything, concerns you about losing weight?"* *"Do you have any concerns about achieving good diabetic control or about hypoglycemic episodes?"*	Benefits about dieting and weight loss *"Tell me what you understand about the benefits of achieving good diabetic control."* *"How would your family respond if you were to lower your Hb A1c?"*

Reasons to Stay the Same (Cons)	Reasons to Change (Pros)
Benefits of nonadherence [b] Less work for spouse preparing family meals Less work in checking glucose levels Relieve stress by eating candy	Concerns about nonadherence Family nags me to look after myself better Risk of hospitalizations Eye, kidney and feet complications
Concerns about adherence Extra costs Hypoglycemic episodes Interferes with work	Benefits of adherence Improve health Live longer Keep my heart in good shape
Resistance	Motivation

Explaining and Obtaining Resistance and Motivation Scores
"The left-hand column represents your reasons to stay the same (resistance to change). The right-hand column represents your reasons to change (motivation to change). On a scale of 0 to 10, 0 meaning none and 10 meaning very high, what score would you give for your reasons to stay the same? [pointing to the left column] *And what score would you give for your reasons to change? Are your resistance and motivation scores based on what you think or feel about change? Now, how would you score your resistance and motivation based on what you feel or think?*

Assessing Motives
"What would persuade you to take better care of your diabetes (or try to lower your Hb A1c, or any other specific aspect of self-care of diabetes)?" [Let patient respond; if necessary, prompt the patient.] *"Would you do it because family and friends wanted you to? Would you do it because you felt that you ought to take better care of your diabetes for your health or any other reason? Would you do it because it is important to you? Or, perhaps for a combination of reasons? Which is most important?"*

Assessing Competing Priorities and Energy
"What competing priorities do you face in taking care of your diabetes?" *"On a scale of zero to ten, how much energy can you put into taking better care of your diabetes?"*

Assessing Confidence and Ability (self-efficacy)
"On a scale of zero to ten, how would you rate your confidence to keep your hemoglobin A1c within normal range (or deal with any other aspect of diabetic self-care)?"   *"On a scale of zero to ten, how would you rate your ability to keep your hemoglobin A1c within normal range (or deal with any other aspect of diabetic self-care)?"*

Assessing Supports
"Would you like others to help you with your diabetes? Who or what could help your diabetes? Do you know of any community programs you can attend to help your diabetes?"
Assessing Barriers
"Do you have difficulties in getting the care that you need?"   *"Do you have money problems that make it difficult for you look after your diabetes?"*   *"Are there people around you who make it more difficult for you to deal with your diabetes?"*

STEP 4: ENHANCING MUTUAL UNDERSTANDING

A. Educate Patients about Health Behavior Change

Practitioner-centered Education
Authoritarian advice-giving (limited applications): State in a firm tone of voice: *"I think you should lose weight, keep to the diabetic diet, check your blood glucose regularly, and keep your blood glucose levels normal with your insulin regimen so that you can reduce your risk of going blind and developing kidney failure."*   Authoritative advice-giving: *"Checking your blood sugar at home helps you know if your levels are normal, but the Hb A1c is the best way to know whether you are keeping good control of your diabetes. If you keep your Hb A1c at normal levels, you can reduce your chance of:*   • *Eye damage (retinopathy) by 76%;*   • *Progression of eye damage (retinopathy) by 54% (proliferative or severe nonproliferative retinopathy by 47%);*   • *Protein in your urine (microalbuminuria: > 40 mg per 24 hours by 39% and > 300 micrograms per 24 hours by 54%);*   • *Nerve damage (neuropathy) by 60%.*   *But tight control of your blood glucose (intensive insulin therapy) may cause a two- to three-fold increase in severe hypoglycemia."*

Patient-centered Education about Risks and Harm
Risk of diabetic complications: *"At the moment, you are not noticing any problems with your diabetes, but are you aware of the problems?"* [Let patient respond, and then provide additional information that you think the patient is most interested in hearing.] *"Unfortunately, it can damage your (eyes, kidneys, feet, nerves, and heart) without your being aware of it until it causes symptoms years later. The way to reduce your risk of complications is to check your Hb A1c on a regular basis. Are you willing to have this blood test every three months or so?"* Complications of diabetes: *"What concerns do you have about your health?"* [Let patient respond.] *"I'm concerned that your diabetes is causing eye damage (or any other complication needing specialist care) and that it will progress unless you see the eye doctor."*

Family-centered Education
Family-centered advice-giving: *"You and your family both know that high sugar levels put you at risk for complications and increase your risk of dying. You seem to be willing to accept the fact you may die from diabetic complications."* [Pause and let patient respond. Assuming an affirmative response, continue.] *"But your family doesn't seem ready for you to die, and they want to help reduce your risk of complications. How about you and your family working together to avoid diabetic complications so that you can maintain your quality of life before you die?"*

B. Use Nondirect Interventions to Lower Patient Resistance

Use simple reflection to elicit ambivalence: *"Keeping to the diet (losing weight or checking your blood glucose) regularly is difficult. You feel well even when your blood glucose is high."*
Probe priorities to explore ambivalence: *"In what ways is your life easier by not keeping your diabetes under tight control?"*   *"This may seem an unusual request, but take a moment to think about the most important benefit of not sticking strictly to the diabetic recommendations."* [Pause for silence; if necessary, ask:] *"What is it?"*   *"What concerns you most about not keeping your hemoglobin A1c within normal range?"*   *"What would concern you most if you tried harder to control your weight, blood glucose, and/or diabetes? What are the most important benefits of controlling your diabetes?"*
Use double-sided reflection to summarize ambivalence: *"On the one hand, if you achieve normal glucose levels you will reduce your risk of complications, but on the other hand, you are more likely to have hypoglycemic attacks."*
Acknowledge ambivalence: *"People often have mixed feelings about not keeping strictly to the diabetic diet."*   *"People often have mixed feelings about not following the recommendations."*
Emphasize personal responsibility and choice (useful when patients are being resistant): *"Whether you decide to try and keep your hemoglobin A1c within the normal range is up to you, but I'm willing to help you prevent diabetic complications."*
Explore the future questioning: *"What was your diabetes like a few years ago, what is it like now, and what do you think it will be like in five to ten years?"*

C. Use Direct Interventions to Motivate Patient Change

Back-to-the-future Questioning
"If you developed a diabetic complication now, would you try to keep your diabetes in better control in the future?" [Provided that the patient shows some interest in prevention, continue.] *"Do you want to wait and see if you develop a complication before deciding to change?"* [If the patient remains interested in prevention, continue.] *"What would it take for you to decide to take better control of your diabetes?"* [If the patient is ambivalent or not interested in prevention, ask:] *"Can you share with me what is difficult about changing?"*

Benefit Substitution
"Are there ways for you to enjoy your food, but at the same time stay within the dietary recommendations or simply reduce the amount that you eat? For example, when you overeat on some occasions, can you check your glucose levels before such an occasion and give yourself some extra regular insulin?"

Clarifying Values
Questions that probe values: *"What is more important in your life than trying to prevent the complications of diabetes?"* Questions that contrast values: *"Is eating regular meals with your family more important to you than trying to avoid the long-term complications of diabetes?"* *"Is being a parent and spouse more important to you than trying to avoid the long-term complications of diabetes?"* Questions that contrast values and behavior: *"If you say that your health is more important than eating regular meals with your family, you're saying one thing and doing another. What would convince you to do what you say?"*

Challenging Rationalizations
"May I propose a few things that might help you think about your diabetes differently?" [With an affirmative response from the patient, continue.] *"It may make you pause and think about how much effort you want to put into preventing complications. You don't have to say anything if you don't feel like it, and if you want me to stop talking about diabetes, just tell me."* [Choose any of the following questions and, if necessary, prompt with a follow-up comment] *"Some diabetics don't think that they will ever get any complications, but later regret that they did not take better care of themselves."* *"Diabetes is deceptive. It makes you think that you do not have a disease because you can feel so well. But, by the time you develop symptoms, the damage is often done and difficult to reverse."* *"Many people say that they have to die sometime from something, so they live as they please for now and don't have any concerns about dying or the quality of their life before they die."* *"Your blood glucose levels are good when you check them at home, but your Hb A1c is still high."* [These statements help patients to reexamine their rationalizations for not changing]

Discrepancies
Identify discrepancies between a behavior and self-interest: *"You say that you want to stay well, but your increased level of Hb A1c is putting you at risk of diabetic complications."* Identify differences in motivational reasons: *"What would it take for you to care for yourself in terms of taking the tablets and sticking to the diet in the same way that you look after your feet?"*

176

Reframing Items, Issues or Events
Change a reason not to adhere into a reason to adhere: *"Although you can have high blood glucose levels and feel well, it still puts you at high risk for developing complications."* Enhance a reason to adhere to diabetic recommendations: *"Your spouse nags you about not sticking to your diet, but could this show how much he or she is really concerned about your health?"* Diminish a reason not to adhere: *"You say that you enjoy eating out with your friends, but can you enjoy your friends and also stick to your diet?"*

Amplified Reflection
"So, you're not worried at all about diabetic complications?" *"So, you believe that you are in some way specially protected from the complications of diabetes."*

Differences in Motivational Reasons
"You put so much effort into taking great care of your family, but what would it take for you to put more effort into taking care of your diabetes?" *"You regularly check your feet because you do not want to have any more ulcers* [integrated motivation]. *You feel that you ought to take medication* [introjected motivation]. *You check your blood glucose levels when your spouse prompts you to* [extrinsic motivation], *but you don't seem at all concerned about sticking to your diet* [indifferent motivation]. *What would it take for you to lower your Hb A1c as much as possible in the same way that you look after your feet?"*

Monitoring Changes in Resistance and Motivation Scores
"What scores would you now give for your resistance and motivation, using the scale of 0-10?" "Why did you change your resistance score? And why did you change your motivation score?" "You can learn a lot about yourself even if your scores got worse and went in the wrong direction. Sometimes it helps if your resistance score goes up and your motivation score goes down because this can teach you what it would take to change for good."

D. Clarify Differences in Perception about Patient Self-efficacy

Confidence and Ability (self-efficacy)
"On a scale of zero to ten, how would you now rate your ability to lower your Hb A1c (or any other self-care task for diabetes)? And how would your rate your confidence to lower your Hb A1c to below 7?" [Let patient respond; address whether you agree with your patient's self-assessment.]

STEP 5: IMPLEMENTING A PLAN FOR CHANGE

Clarifying Persistent Differences in Perceptions
"I think it is important for us to be clear about whether we see the benefits, risks, and harm the same way or differently because that will affect how we work together. I understand what you like about eating whatever you want, but I seem to be more concerned about the risks and harm caused by your poor diabetic control than you are. What do you think?"

A. Evaluate Patient Commitment toward a Plan of Change

Competing Priorities
"What is going on in your life that makes it difficult for you to take better care of your diabetes? And anything else?"
"What would it take for you to put good diabetic care at the top of your list of things to do?"
Or, *"What is stopping you from putting good diabetic care at the top of your list of things to do?"*

Energy
"What is going on that makes it difficult for you to devote your energy to taking better care of your diabetes?"
"What would it take for you to put your energy into taking better care of your diabetes?"
"If you don't have any energy to change, what would it take for you to get your energy back?"

Motives
"What makes you commit yourself to this change? And what else?"
"You say that you are here because your spouse wanted you to come, but what would it take for you to come for your own reasons?"

B. Decide about Goals for Change

Range of Goals for Improving Self-care of Diabetes

Think about change
    Think more about what it would take to achieve normal Hb A1c
    Use a decision balance to address any behavior change issues
Prepare for change
    Plan how to take better care of diabetes
    Learn about managing diabetic complications
    Involve family and friends in plans to change
Take action
    Set a change date to change behavior or address any diabetic issues
Additional goals
    Referral to specialists
    Referral to community resources

C. Work toward Solutions (incorporating MED-STAT)[1]

Interventions	Solution-based Language for Behavior Change[1]
Miracle question (explore change)	*"Suppose a miracle happened, and you lost 15-20 pounds in a year so that you could stop taking diabetic tablets. What would your life be like then? How would you and your family respond?"*
Exceptions (identify strengths)	*"How did you stop yourself from overeating on an occasion when you felt depressed?"*
Differences (use strengths)	*"How does this occasion compare to other situations when you felt depressed and overate?"*
Scaling (assess motivation, self-efficacy and outcome expectancy)	*"On a scale of zero to ten, how would you score your (motivation, competence, and confidence) to keep to a diabetic recommendation (lose weight, keep to a diet, maintain weight loss, and/or normalize your Hb A1c)?"* *"How would you rate whether you can achieve your goal for change (outcome expectancy)?"* *"Was there a time when your scores were higher than now? What would increase your scores? Can you make a list of that? What would it take to tip the balance in favor of higher scores?"*
Timeouts (consider alternatives)	*"What other ideas do you have about how you could handle depression and diabetes better? What would it take for you to put those ideas into practice?"*
Accolades (enhance efficacy)	*"You managed to keep your Hb A1c below nine most of the time, but how could you build on what you are doing right to do better still?"*
Task appraisals (encourage action)	*"What would it take for you to keep your Hb A1c as low as possible?"*

STEP 6: FOLLOWING THROUGH

Arranging Follow-up

Providing Rationale and Purpose for Follow-up

"I think a follow-up would be important in order for us to [choose one or more of the following]:
     Check up on your Hb A1c;
     Monitor for complications;
     Provide care for the complications." [and then make a follow-up appointment.]

Clarifying Patients' Reasons to Attend Follow-up
"What do you understand as your reasons for your attending a follow-up appointment? What is important for you to address at the next appointment?"
Timing, Duration and Frequency of Follow-up Appointments
"How often do you think you should come back to see me?"   *"I think it's important for you to decide when to come back for a follow-up appointment. I will certainly share what I think about this, but I'm more interested in what* you *think."*

Use Methods to Ensure Change and Prevent Relapse

A diary to track change:

"Are you interested in keeping a diary to understand your diabetes better so that you can anticipate when you are likely to relapse from good diabetic control? It would also help if you were to record your thoughts and feelings during situations when you feel tempted to relapse."

Relapse prevention:

Management of risk situations: *"Which kind of situations will make it difficult for you to keep to your goals for good diabetic control? What ways can you deal with those difficulties?"*

Pharmacological management: *"What difficulties do you have in taking your tablets on a regular basis? Do you feel that you know how to alter your insulin dose according to blood glucose readings and meal sizes?"*

Emotional management: *"When you feel upset [or any other negative emotions], how do you deal with those feelings instead of eating?"*

Reevaluation of supports: *"Would it help to have someone to help you work toward your goal of change?"*

Reevaluation of barriers: *"What do you think is making it difficult for you to maintain your goal for change? How do you think you're going to handle those situations?"*

Use of positive reinforcement: *"Would rewards help you keep to your goals for change? What would those be?"*

Motivational reevaluation:

"Let's look again at your motivational balance and talk about whether you still think your reasons to change are really more important than your reasons to stay the same. This may help you stick to the diabetic recommendations when you have difficulties in keeping to them."

Endnotes

a. During the course of chronic diabetes, practitioners, patients, and families have different perceptions and priorities about the need to address adherence and the goal of achieving normoglycemia. They often have different levels of investment in addressing these issues and are therefore at different stages in terms of their readiness to address any aspect of adherence to self-care of diabetes. When this occurs, practitioners, patients, and families usually experience resistance in working together. To avoid this, they can collaborate in ways that help them begin to work through the stages of change together.

To work toward this goal, practitioners can use their agenda-setting skills to help patients and family members become more willing to discuss, think about, and address the multiple issues related to self-care of diabetes. Practitioners also can conduct the agenda-setting phase in ways that help patients and families change their priorities so that patients become more activate in their self-care of diabetes.

In addition to practitioners, patients, and families having different agendas and priorities in dealing with multiple issues, they often perceive the benefits of and concerns about nonadherence or adherence to a diabetic regimen differently. Patients often change their perceptions over time about preventive issues. For example, some patients are least motivated to adhere to their self-care regimen during the phase of primary prevention because they feel relatively well and rarely suffer any ill consequences from complications; they may become more motivated to change when early complications occur.

b. Benefits to patients of suboptimal self-care.

Lifestyle: *"I save money by not taking the tablets." "I don't want to cause any inconvenience to my family by sticking to the diet." "The diabetic diet makes extra work for my spouse." "The diet (Chemstrip, etc.) is expensive." "The diet creates a lot of extra work."*

Affective (mood-enhancing or mood-diminishing): *"Eating is pleasurable and makes me feel good." "Eating helps relieve my stress/anxiety."*

Psychological coping: *"Ignoring diabetes is a way to avoid thinking about what might happen to me." "I have too much stress in my life to keep on top of diabetes." "It is impossible for me to look after number one and keep on top of diabetes as a single parent looking after three children."*

Social coping: *"Diabetes interferes with my social life, like going to parties." "My friends don't understand what it is like living with diabetes, so it is easier to eat and drink just like them."*

Spiritual coping: *"I am not afraid of death, so why should I worry about dealing with diabetes?"*

Reference List

1. Giorlando ME, Schilling RJ. On becoming a solution-focused physician: The MED-STAT acronym. Families, Systems & Health 1997;15: 361-373

AFTERWORD

Patients with unhealthy behaviors are locked in rooms without a key to escape. Each room has a different key. Your dialogue with patients can cut a key to open the door to the possibility of change. Yet, many patients still get stuck at the door's threshold. Your ongoing dialogue can help patients cross the threshold. In other words, your dialogue can help them de-program their unhealthy habit (unlock the door) and re-program it into a healthy one (cross the threshold). This art of dialogue is a lifelong learning process.

Such lifelong learning involves using the four phases of the CPD model: self-focused, method-focused, learner-centered and patient-centered methods. These methods can enhance your skills at motivating behavior change throughout your professional career. The six-step approach provides you with ways of initiating dialogues with patients in new ways. The motivational principles (listed in Chapter 1, Book 1) can help you overcome awkward moments, impasses, missed opportunities and/or "branch points" arising from your interactions with patients; you can also use the PARE improvement cycle to address these specific situations so that you become increasingly more effective in working with your patients. This journey of professional enrichment is without end.

APPENDIX A: CHECKLISTS FOR REVIEWING A VIDEO DEMONSTRATION

You can assess your level of understanding about some micro skills before and after watching a video demonstration. An example of three sequential tasks will illustrate how you can use a method-centered approach to understand a limited range of micro skills:

- Clarify a patient's issues about change
- Lower patient resistance
- Enhance patient motivation

The tasks on the next three pages describes the micro skills for completing these tasks, using tobacco as an example. You can watch a demonstration of these three tasks on CD-ROM, videotape and the Web site www.MotivateHealthyhabits.com. After watching the three tasks, you can use the 0-10 scale to assess whether this demonstration helped you to increase your level of understanding about the micro skills used in each step, from before to after watching the videotape

Task 1: Clarify a patient's issues about change

Ask about Readiness to Change
"Where are you in terms of your smoking?" [Select one] *"Are you really not thinking about changing?" "Are you thinking about it?" "Are you willing to make a change?"*

Provide a Stage-specific Rationale and Gain Consent to Use the Decision Balance
Precontemplation: *"You just told me that you are just not interested in quitting. Would you mind if we did a decision balance together so I can understand better why you want to smoke?"*
Contemplation: *"You told me that you are thinking about quitting. Would you mind if we did a decision balance together? It can help you think more about whether to quit."*
Preparation: *"You're thinking about setting a quit date. Would you mind if we did a decision balance together? It can help you decide on a quit date."*

Show the Decision Balance to the Patient
"Let me show you what a decision balance looks like. You will understand what it is as we go through using it. First, I would like you to list as many benefits as possible that you get from smoking cigarettes. Is it okay to use this decision balance?"

Draw a Decision Balance for the Patient and Ask These Questions	
1. Benefits of smoking *"What do you like about smoking? And what else?"*	*2. Concerns about smoking* *"What, if anything, concerns you about the effects of smoking on your health?"*
3. Concerns about quitting *"Do you have any concerns if you were to quit?"*	*4. Benefits of quitting* *"How do you think your health would improve if you were to quit?"*

Explain and Obtain "Think" and "Feeling" Scores for Resistance and Motivation
"The left column represents your reasons to stay the same (resistance). The right column represents your reasons to change (motivation). On a scale of 0 to 10, 0 meaning none and 10 meaning very high, what score would you give for your reasons to stay the same? [pointing to the left column] And what score would you give for your reasons to change? Are your resistance and motivation scores based on what you think or feel about change? Now, how would you score your resistance and motivation based on what you feel or think?"

Assess Your Level of Understanding in Using These Micro Skills	Before	After
1. Assessing the patient's readiness to change		
2. Providing an appropriate rationale for using a decision balance		
3. Showing the patient what the decision balance looks like		
4. Itemizing the benefits of the risk behavior		
5. Itemizing the concerns about the risk behavior		
6. Itemized the concerns about adopting a healthy behavior		
7. Itemized the benefits of adopting a healthy behavior		
8. Explained resistance and motivation scores		
9. Obtained "think" and "feeling" scores for resistance and motivation		
10. Gave the decision balance back to the patient		

Task 2: Lower patient resistance

Assess Impact of Using Nondirect Interventions Using the 0-10 Scale		Score
Use simple reflection: *"So, smoking smoothes your nerves?"* *"...helps you think clearer if you quit?"*		
Probe priorities: *"Which is the most important reason to smoke? And what about the most important reason to think about quitting?"*		
Use double-sided reflection: *"On the one hand, smoking helps you relax, but, on the other hand, you are concerned about the effects of smoking on your son's health."*		
Explore the future: *"What do you think is going to happen to your health in the future if you continue smoking over the next 5-10 years?"*		
Acknowledge ambivalence: *"So it makes you have some mixed feelings about smoking?"*		
Emphasize personal responsibility and choice: *"It's really up to you to decide whether to think about your smoking and quitting."*		
Guess what her resistance score is now	**Guess what her motivation score is now**	

Which interventions had the greatest impact on the patient, and why?
Give your reasons for guessing whether you think that the patient changed her scores, or not.
Now watch the videotape and see what the patient thinks.

Assess Your Level of Understanding in Using These Micro Skills	Before	After
Probe priorities		
Use double-sided reflection		
Explore the future		
Acknowledge ambivalence		
Emphasize personal responsibility and choice		
Use simple reflection		

Task 3: Enhance patient motivation

Assess Impact of Using Direct Interventions Using the 0-10 Scale			Score
Use benefit substitution: *"I'm just wondering if there are some other ways that you could soothe your nerves?"*			
Bring the future to the present: *"Imagine that you developed a health problem caused by smoking sometime in the future. Suppose that happened now; what would you do?"*			
Clarify values: *"What is more important to you – smoking to relax or your son's health?"*			
Identify discrepancies: *"But you are saying one thing and doing another."*			
Use differences in motivational reasons: *"I am just wondering if you could take the energy that you use to protect your son's health and protect your own health as well?"*			
Reframe events or issues: *"You say that smoking helps you relax but it's really just a sign of nicotine addiction."*			
Guess what her resistance score is now		**Guess what her motivation score is now**	

Which interventions had the greatest impact on the patient, and why?
Give your reasons for guessing whether you think that the patient changed her scores, or not.
Now watch the videotape and see what the patient thinks.

Assess Your Level of Understanding in Using These Micro Skills	Before	After
Use back-to-the-future questioning		
Use benefit substitution		
Clarify values		
Use discrepancies		
Reframe items, issues or events		
Use differences in motivational reasons		

A method-focused approach can appear unnatural, because the demonstration is following a script for developing micro skills. If you replicate this demonstration with a real patient, you are practicing specific skills out of context.

To practice using these skills, you need to obtain patients' consent and inform them that this is a learning opportunity for you. In following such a script, you may feel constrained by this learning process because you may want to follow the patient's lead and address issues outside of the script: in other words, be patient-centered. If you do what you usually do, however, you are not learning anything new.

The goal of using a method-centered approach is to first expand your range and depth of skills so that you can learn how to be effectively patient-centered. Such practice sessions, however, do not guarantee that you can use these micro skills equally well, or use them in a highly individualized manner with patients. To move beyond being method-focused, you need to use learner-centered and patient-centered training approaches.

After watching these demonstrations, you can try and use these micro skills in practice sessions and use the checklists in Worksheets 1.6 and 1.7 to assess any changes in your level of competence

APPENDIX B: CHECKLISTS FOR PRACTICING MICRO SKILLS

Working with a colleague (or simulated patient) in role plays can help you enhance your skills. One person can play the "practitioner" role, and the other can play the "patient" role. You both stay in the same role throughout the three tasks listed below. The "patient" selects a risk behavior and fills out a decision balance with at least two items in each of the four quadrants (see chart below) before the practice session. Because the items in the quadrants will be compared to those of the "practitioner" in Tasks 2 and 3, the "patient" should not show the fully itemized decision balance to the "practitioner" until after Task 1 is completed. In this particular exercise, smoking is the risk behavior selected.

Example of a Decision Balance

Reasons to stay the same	*Reasons to change*
1. What are the benefits of your risk behavior?	*2. What concerns do you have about your risk behavior?*
3. What concerns do you have if you were to change?	*4. What are the benefits of changing?*

The "practitioner" completes the tasks listed below.

- Task 1: Clarify Issues About Change
  Use a decision balance and list at least two items for each quadrant
- Task 2: Lower Patient Resistance
  Select in advance and use at least two nondirect interventions
- Task 3: Enhance Patient Motivation
  Select in advance and use at least two direct interventions

After completing Task 1, the "patient" gives the fully itemized decision balance to the "practitioner" so that he or she has more information to use when selecting the nondirect and direct interventions that he or she thinks will be most effective. It is better for the "practitioner" to use two such interventions well rather than to rush through three or more. You (the "practitioner") also will make the most of these learning opportunities if you try options that do not come naturally to you. For example, you may have a need to learn how to use nondirect interventions because you may have a natural ability to be direct with patients. Or, the converse may be true for you. Sometimes, a poorly implemented intervention has a greater impact than a well-delivered one. Both the "practitioner" and "patient" then fill out a checklist for each task to reflect about their shared experience and to compare perceptions about the interaction.

The work plan with a suggested timetable (see below) is a guide for developing new skills. This timetable is a calculated to provide a rapid learning opportunity about how to work with patients in new ways. Any additional time you could spend would be beneficial for learning the skill.

Work Plan and Suggested Timetable for Task 1	**Minutes**
1. Study the one-page handout and evaluation checklist for the task	5
2. Role-play and complete the task	6
3. Fill out the checklist for the task	3
4. Debriefing: discuss differences between your checklists and between your questionnaire	6
Total time for one task	20
5. Repeat the same format for Tasks 2 and 3. Total time for 3 tasks	60

The format for debriefing after each task is:

- Look for any differences between your checklists and your scores. Do not alter your responses. It is an issue about understanding your differences for learning purposes, not about being right or wrong. Your differences in perceptions about a shared experience provide the greatest learning opportunities. Now, discuss your differences in responses. What did you learn from your differences?
- The "practitioner" evaluates only those interventions that were selected and used in Tasks 2 and 3. The "patient," however, can respond to all the statements on the checklist because the interventions can have a secondary impact beyond their primary intentions. The reason for the "patient" to fill out the whole checklist is because motivational interventions can have linear (primary) and nonlinear (secondary) impacts. For example, in practice you may ask a patient to generate a list of benefits for smoking, but this question may make the patient think profoundly about values concerning health, disease, and smoking and its impact on his or her children. In other words, the secondary impact can be greater than its primary intention. Now, ask the "patient" why his or her scores were higher or lower than your scores on the interventions used.
- The "practitioner," observers, and the "patient" each identify an additional aspect of the interaction that was done well but not identified during the discussion of Tasks 2 and 3. In addition, you can identify areas for improvement. This learning process can enhance your ability for reflection-in-action more effectively: in other words, how to handle awkward moments, branch points, or stuck moments as they arise. The feedback guidelines described Chapter 2 (page 37) can also help you when working with a colleague or in small group.

In addition, you can videotape (or audiotape) your role plays for in-depth reflection. For group sessions, the following guidelines for the participants and the "patient" for videotape (and audiotape) reviews can enhance the learning process: Tasks for the "practitioner" (presenter).

The presenter has the remote control and can stop the tape at any time to identify two things that were done well and two things that could be improved. In addition, the presenter can:

- Request feedback from the observers and the "patient" about what happened
- Ask the "patient" about how something affected him or her
- Check if the "patient" agrees with the presenter's self-assessment

Tasks for group participants and the "patient"

Each person is expected to stop the tape to identify one thing that was done well. During these pauses, a question can be more effective than making a statement or comment.

For example, rather than saying: *"You made the 'patient' feel uncomfortable,"* ask the presenter, *"How do you think the 'patient' felt at that moment?"* Then ask the "patient," *"How did you feel at that moment?"*

You can download the handouts (on the next 9 pages) from the Web site: www.MotivateHealthyHabits.com.

Task 1 for Practitioner—Clarify issues about change using a decision balance

Ask about Readiness to Change
"Where are you in terms of your smoking?" [Select one or more of these questions] *"Are you really not thinking about changing?" "Are you thinking about it?" "Are you willing to make a change?"*
Provide a Stage-specific Rationale and Gain Consent to Use the Decision Balance
Precontemplation: *"You just told me that you are just not interested in quitting. Would you mind if we did a decision balance together? It can help me better understand why you do not want to quit."*
Contemplation: *"You told me that you are thinking about quitting. Would you mind if we did a decision balance together? It can help you think more about whether to quit."*
Preparation: *"You're thinking about setting a quit date. Would you mind if we did a decision balance together? It can help you decide on a quit date."*
Show the Decision Balance to the Patient
"Let me show you what a decision balance looks like. You will understand what it is as we go through using it. First, I would like you to list as many benefits as possible that you get from smoking cigarettes. Is it okay to use this decision balance?"

Draw a Decision Balance for the Patient and Ask These Questions	
1. Benefits of smoking *"What do you like about smoking? And what else?"*	*2. Concerns about smoking* *"What, if anything, concerns you about the effects of smoking on your health?"*
3. Concerns about quitting *"Do you have any concerns if you were to quit?"*	*4. Benefits of quitting* *"How do you think your health would improve if you were to quit?"*

Explain and Obtain "Think" and "Feeling" Scores for Resistance and Motivation
"The left column represents your reasons to stay the same (resistance). The right column represents your reasons to change (motivation). On a scale of 0 to 10, 0 meaning none and 10 meaning very high, what score would you give for your reasons to stay the same? [pointing to the left column] And what score would you give for your reasons to change? Are your resistance and motivation scores based on what you think or feel about change? Now, how would you score your resistance and motivation based on what you feel or think?"

Practitioner Checklist for Task 1—Assess Your Competence and Patient Impact

Assess your level of competence using the 0-10 scale:

0	1	2	3	4	5	6	7	8	9	10
Not done	*Low*				*Average*					*Excellent*

A self-assessment	Score
1. Assessed the patient's readiness to change	
2. Provided the patient with an appropriate rationale for using a decision balance	
3. Showed the patient what the decision balance looks like	
4. Itemized at least two benefits of the risk behavior	
5. Itemized at least two concerns about the risk behavior	
6. Itemized at least two concerns about adopting a healthy behavior	
7. Itemized at least two benefits of adopting a healthy behavior	
8. Explained resistance and motivation scores	
9. Obtained "think" and "feeling" scores for resistance and motivation	
10. Gave the decision balance back to the patient	

Assess your impact on your patient (using the 0-10 scale) by giving your opinion about the following statements:

0	1	2	3	4	5	6	7	8	9	10
Feel neutral		*Slightly agree*			*Moderately agree*				*Strongly agree*	

Your perception about your impact on the patient	Score
I provided an effective rationale for using the decision balance to the patient.	
I showed the decision balance to the patient and helped him or her understand it by using it.	
I gave a good explanation to the patient about how to rate his or her resistance and motivation.	
The decision balance helped my patient understand more about change.	
My patient wanted to keep the decision balance.	

Now look at your patient's form to clarify the reasons for any differences. Ask your patient questions about why your scores differ. Please do not change your checklist after discussing your differences.

Patient Checklist for Task 1:
Assessing Your Practitioner's Competence and Impact

Assess your practitioner's level of competence, using the 0-10 scale:

0	1	2	3	4	5	6	7	8	9	10
Not done	*Low*				*Average*					*Excellent*

Assessment of my practitioner's competence in doing the following:	Score
1. Assessed my readiness to change	
2. Provided me with an appropriate rationale for using a decision balance	
3. Showed me what the decision balance looks like	
4. Itemized at least two benefits of the risk behavior	
5. Itemized at least two concerns about the risk behavior	
6. Itemized at least two concerns about adopting a healthy behavior	
7. Itemized at least two benefits of adopting a healthy behavior	
8. Explained resistance and motivation scores	
9. Obtained "think" and "feeling" scores for resistance and motivation	
10. Gave the decision balance back to me	

Assess your practitioner's impact on you (using the 0-10 scale) by giving your opinion about the following statements:

0	1	2	3	4	5	6	7	8	9	10
Feel neutral		*Slightly agree*			*Moderately agree*				*Strongly agree*	

Your perception about your practitioner's impact on you	Score
My practitioner provided an effective rationale for using the decision balance.	
My practitioner showed me the decision balance and helped me understand it by using it.	
My practitioner gave me a good explanation about how to rate my resistance and motivation.	
The decision balance helped me think more about change.	
My practitioner gave me the decision balance in a way that I wanted to keep it.	

Now look at your practitioner's form. Let your practitioner ask questions about any differences in scores. Please do not change your checklist after discussing your differences.

Task 2 for Practitioner—Lower Patient Resistance Using Nondirect Interventions

Explain to Patient What You Are Trying to Do
"I'd like to better understand why you do not want (are reluctant, or are finding it difficult) to change. This may help you to change your resistance and motivation scores."
Select Two or More Nondirect Interventions to Practice with Your Patient
Probe priorities to explore ambivalence: *"So, what is the most important reason for you to smoke? And what is the most important reason for you to quit?"*
Use double-sided reflection to summarize ambivalence: *"On the one hand, you said that smoking helps you relieve your stress, but, on the other hand, you are concerned about how smoking stresses your heart."*
Use explore-the-future questioning: *"So, what was your heart like five years ago when you were smoking, compared to now? What do you think your heart will be like in five years?"*
Acknowledge ambivalence to validate patient's experience: *"You seem to have mixed feelings about your smoking. You smoke to relax from the stresses of being a single parent, but you are concerned about its effects on your children at home."*
Emphasize personal responsibility and choice (useful when the patient is being resistant): *"What you decide to do about smoking is entirely up to you, but I'll help you if you would like me to."*
Use simple reflection to elicit ambivalence: *"So, smoking helps to relieve your stress."*
Ask Patient Whether His or Her Resistance and Motivation Scores Have Now Changed

Practitioner Checklist for Task 2: Assessing the Impact of Nondirect Interventions

Give a score only to those interventions that you used.

To what extent do you agree with these statements, using the 0-10 scale?	Score
I helped my patient better understand his or her priorities about change. *(Probed priorities to explore ambivalence)*	
Doubled-sided reflection helped my patient think more about ambivalence. *(Used double-sided reflection to summarize ambivalence)*	
I helped my patient think more about his or her risk behavior and future health. *(Used explore-the-future questioning)*	
Acknowledging my patient's ambivalence helped him or her feel better understood. *(Acknowledged ambivalence)*	
I helped my patient better understand his or her responsibility about making a change. *(Emphasized personal responsibility and choice)*	
I helped my patient better understand: a) the benefits of risk behavior.	
b) concerns about risk behavior.	
c) concerns about changing.	
d) the benefits of changing. *(Used simple reflection to understand the patient better)*	
I helped my patient to reassess his or her resistance and motivation scores.	

Ask your patient questions about why your scores differ, and why he or she changed his or her resistance and motivation scores.

Patient Checklist for Task 2: Assessing the Impact of Nondirect Interventions

Give a score for each of the statements below, even though your practitioner only used 2-3 interventions.

To what extent do you agree with these statements, using the 0-10 scale?	Score
My practitioner helped me better understand my priorities about change. *(Probed priorities to explore ambivalence)*	
My practitioner's use of doubled-sided reflection helped me think more about ambivalence. *(Used double-sided reflection to summarize ambivalence)*	
My practitioner helped me think more about my risk behavior and future health. *(Used explore-the-future questioning)*	
My practitioner's acknowledgment of my ambivalence helped me feel more understood. *(Acknowledged ambivalence)*	
My practitioner helped me better understand my responsibility about making a change. *(Emphasized personal responsibility and choice)*	
My practitioner helped me better understand: a) the benefits of my risk behavior.	
b) my concerns about my risk behavior.	
c) my concerns about changing.	
d) the benefits of my changing. *(Used simple reflection to understand me better.)*	
My practitioner helped me reassess my resistance and motivation scores.	

Let your practitioner ask questions about any differences in scores, and be prepared to explain why you changed your resistance and motivation scores.

Task 3 for Practitioner—Enhance Patient Motivation Using Direct Interventions

Explain to Patient What You Are Trying to Do
"I would like to see if I can help you increase your motivation scores. After I have tried to help you, I'll ask you again what your resistance and motivation scores are to see if they have changed."
Select Two or More Direct Interventions to Practice with Your Patient
Use back-to-the-future questioning: *"If you had a heart attack now, would you quit smoking?"* [Provided that the patient shows some interest in prevention, continue.] *"Do you want to wait and see if this happens before deciding to quit?"* [If the patient remains interested in prevention, continue.] *"What would really convince you to quit?"* [If the patient is ambivalent, or not interested in prevention, ask] *"Would you mind sharing with me why you don't want to quit?"*
Use benefit substitution: *"In what kind of stressful situations do you smoke?"* *"How can you relieve your stress instead of smoking?"* *"Could you write down four or five ways of relieving stress for each situation and bring the list in next time?"*
Clarify values: *"So, what is more important in your life than smoking? Is smoking and reducing your stress more important to you than your heart? If you say that your health is more important than smoking, you're saying one thing and doing another. What would convince you to do what you say?"*
Use discrepancies: *"You say that smoking relieves your stress."* [Let patient acknowledge your comments nonverbally.] *"But it also stresses your heart and your family because they worry about your health."* [Let patient respond.]
Reframe events, items or issues: *"You say that smoking gives you pleasure, but it makes you feel worse when you smoke too much, and it makes your cough worse in the morning."*
Use differences in motivational reasons: *"What would it take for you to quit smoking and take care of your health in the same way that you take care of your family (or any other activities that the patient is highly motivated to do)?"*
Ask Patient Whether His or Her Resistance and Motivation Scores Have Changed

Practitioner Checklist for Task 3: Assessing the Impact of Direct Interventions

Give a score only to those interventions that you used.

To what extent do you agree with these statements, using the 0-10 scale?	Score
I helped my patient think about what his or her life would be like if he or she developed a future complication now. *(Used back-to-the-future questioning)*	
I helped my patient see that he or she could obtain the benefits from the risk behavior in alternative ways. *(Used benefit substitution)*	
I helped my patient think about values in terms of risk behaviors, health, and other aspects of his or her life. *(Clarified values)*	
I pointed out some discrepancies or differences between what my patient does and what he or she says that made my patient really think about change in new ways. *(Used discrepancies)*	
I helped my patient change his or her perceptions about benefits and concerns on his or her decision balance. *(Reframed events, items or issues)*	
I helped my patient think about how he or she could use motivation to do things well in life and to change behavior. *(Used differences in motivational reasons)*	
I helped my patient to reassess his or her resistance and motivation scores.	

Ask your patient questions about why your scores differ, and why he or she changed his or her resistance and motivation scores.

Patient Checklist for Task 3: Assessing the Impact of Direct Interventions

Give a score for each of the statements below, even though the practitioner only used 2-3 interventions.

To what extent do you agree with these statements, using the 0-10 scale?	Score
My practitioner helped me think about what my life would be like if I developed a future complication now. *(Used back-to-the-future questioning)*	
My practitioner helped me see that I could obtain the benefits from my risk behavior in alternative ways. *(Used benefit substitution)*	
My practitioner helped me think about my values in terms of my risk behavior, my health, and other aspects of my life. *(Clarified values)*	
My practitioner pointed out some discrepancies or differences between what I do and what I say that made me really think about change in new ways. *(Used discrepancies)*	
My practitioner helped me change my perceptions about the benefits and concerns on my decision balance. *(Reframed events, items or issues)*	
My practitioner helped me think about how I could use my motivation to do things well in my life and use it to change my behavior. *(Used differences in motivational reasons)*	
My practitioner helped me to reassess my resistance and motivation scores.	

Let your practitioner ask questions about any differences in scores, and be prepared to explain why you changed your resistance and motivation scores.

APPENDIX C: ASSESSING OVERALL IMPACT OF USING MICRO SKILLS

Patient Questionnaire

Please fill out this questionnaire as honestly as you can. Your practitioner will fill out a similar one. We do not expect your answers to be in 100% agreement. After filling it out, we would like you to share your responses and talk about how you evaluated this experience differently.

1= Strongly disagree 2= Disagree 3= Neither agree or disagree 4= Agree 5= Strongly agree

Keeping in mind what just happened during your encounter, use the scale above to rate whether you agree or disagree with the following:	1	2	3	4	5
My practitioner helped me understand why he or she wanted me to do a decision balance.					
The decision balance helped me think more about quitting and smoking.					
My practitioner helped me understand better how I benefit from smoking cigarettes.					
My practitioner helped me understand better my concerns if I were to quit.					
Overall, my practitioner really understood my reasons for not wanting to quit.					
My practitioner really helped me overcome my reluctance to consider quitting.					
My practitioner helped me think about how I can obtain the benefits of smoking in alternative ways.					
My practitioner helped me think more about my values in terms of smoking and my health.					
My practitioner really helped me think more about how smoking may affect my future health.					
I felt pressured by my practitioner to quit smoking.					
My practitioner made me feel that I ought to quit smoking.					

Before talking to my practitioner today about my smoking, I was:		**After** talking to my practitioner about my smoking today, I will:	
• not thinking about change		• probably not think about change	
• thinking about change		• think more about change	
• preparing to change		• prepare to quit smoking	
• ready to quit smoking		• quit smoking within one week	

203

Practitioner Questionnaire

Please fill out the questionnaire **after** you have completed the interview. Tell the patient you're going to fill out a similar questionnaire so you can compare views on this experience of working together. After debriefing your patient, please respond to the following questions:

1= Strongly disagree 2= Disagree 3= Neither agree or disagree 4= Agree 5= Strongly agree

Keeping in mind what just happened during your encounter, use the scale above to rate whether you agree or disagree with the following:	1	2	3	4	
I helped my patient understand the reason for doing the decision balance.					
The decision balance helped my patient think more about smoking and quitting.					
I helped my patient understand better how he or she benefits from smoking.					
I helped my patient understand better his or her concerns about quitting.					
Overall, I really understood my patient's reasons for not wanting to quit.					
I really helped my patient overcome his or her reluctance to consider quitting.					
I helped my patient think about how he or she can obtain the benefits of smoking in alternative ways.					
I helped my patient think more about my values in terms of smoking and his or her health.					
I really helped my patient think more about how smoking may affect his or her future health.					
I made my patient feel pressured to quit smoking.					
I made my patient feel like he or she ought to quit smoking.					

At the beginning of the encounter, my patient seemed to be:		**At the end** of the encounter, I think my patient will:	
• not thinking about change		• probably not think about change	
• thinking about change		• think more about change	
• preparing to change		• prepare to quit smoking	
• ready to quit smoking		• quit smoking within one week	

APPENDIX D

Tables

Figures

Learning Exercises

Printed in the United States
3730